Overcoming Anxiety Without Fighting it

Dr Tim Cantopher studied at University College, London, and University College Hospital. He trained as a psychiatrist at St James' Hospital, Portsmouth, and St George's, University of London. He has been a member of the Royal College of Psychiatrists since 1983 and was elected fellow of the college in 1999. He worked as a consultant psychiatrist with the Priory Group of Hospitals from 1993 until his retirement from clinical practice in 2015. This is Dr Cantopher's sixth book, and he has published a number of research projects across the field of psychiatry. Dr Cantopher is married with three children.

Other books by Dr Tim Cantopher:

Depressive Illness: The curse of the strong

Stress-related Illness: Advice for people who give too much

Dying for a Drink: All you need to know to beat the booze

Beating Insomnia: Without really trying

Toxic People: Dealing with dysfunctional relationships

Overcoming Anxiety Without Fighting it

DR TIM CANTOPHER

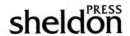

First published in Great Britain in 2019 by Sheldon Press, an imprint of John Murray Press. An Hachette UK company.

2

Copyright © Dr Tim Cantopher 2019

The right of Tim Cantopher to be identified as the Author of the Work has been asserted by him in accordance with the Copyright, Designs and Patents Act 1988.

A CIP catalogue record for this book is available from the British Library.

Paperback ISBN 978 1 84709 498 8

Ebook ISBN 978 1 84709 499 5

Typeset by Cenveo® Publisher Services

Printed and bound in Great Britain by Clays Ltd, Elcograf S.p.A

John Murray Learning policy is to use papers that are natural, renewable and recyclable products and made from wood grown in sustainable forests. The logging and manufacturing processes are expected to conform to the environmental regulations of the country of origin.

Sheldon Press
Carmelite House
50 Victoria Embankment
London EC4Y 0DZ

www.sheldonpress.co.uk

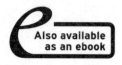

To Laura, who makes me calm in the face of a perplexing world, Hannah, whose bravery and fortitude in the face of anxiety I admire, and Ellen and David, whose serenity in the face of their illnesses is inspirational.

Contents

Acknowledgements

I am grateful to the Royal Society of Medicine for use of their excellent library facilities, my patients for providing any experience and wisdom you may find in these pages, the many researchers and authors whom I have relied on for facts and clinical advice, and my wife for proofreading and giving constructive feedback.

Introduction

I really liked Sally. She was such a good person and I guess she still is. She cared so much about everything and everyone. She tried so hard to make things right and to keep things safe. She moved mountains to get your approval and she expected nothing in return; she didn't seem to feel entitled to much. You didn't have to do much to get on her right side as there wasn't a wrong side with her. She made no judgements about anyone, except about herself – she made plenty of those and they weren't kind. She interpreted harmless comments or gestures as devastating criticisms, as that was what fitted with her view of herself, the world and the future. Sally could never rest, because she was always railing against uncertainty. She saw calamity resulting from every situation, and fear was her constant companion. She needed a lot of reassurance about most things, but somehow it never felt like the reassurance got through. She needed to be sure everything was in control and always safe. It's as if she had gripped life around the throat and couldn't let go, lest it turn around and bite her or those she loved. To her life was a snake, full of danger and venom.

But it's a while since I last saw Sally. From what I hear, her fears and the demands she put on herself made it impossible for her to cope with the world or the people in it. It's no surprise, given the pressure she put on herself and the verbal beating she gave herself every time she felt she got something wrong. Now she's pretty much confined to her flat, where she feels safe from the dangers of the world and the judgements of the people in it. Unfortunately, by avoiding her fears they are growing over time, while her skills and confidence in dealing with day-to-day situations and people are declining. It's difficult to see how she's going to escape the prison she's put herself in.

It's such a shame, as Sally has so much to offer. If only she could believe that, to suspend her judgements on herself for long enough to give her a life.

Tricia is Sally's opposite. Strangely, they were friends until Sally stopped going out, or at least Tricia said they were. Actually, I never saw Tricia do anything for Sally and she seemed to use her for her own convenience, taking advantage of Sally's keenness to please. The thing is, Tricia really doesn't give a damn about anything. She's impulsive, reckless and thoughtless, but then that's part of her charm. She just blows with the wind and her carefree attitude is a breath of fresh air. I wouldn't want to rely on her though, or to get in her way, as she'll just roll right over you and your feelings. Tricia could do with a bit of Sally's fear. As a friend, I'd rather have Sally. If only she could have just a little of Tricia's insouciance. Not too much, just a bit.

Is that possible? Sally has always tended to anxiety, though it is only recently that it has led to her withdrawing from the world. Why does she care so much and live in so much fear? Where do the differences between Sally and Tricia come from? Is there one core difference in the way they see the world which underpins their differences, or maybe several? Were they just made differently, or was it different experiences in their formative years which made them the way they are? How come Sally has changed, that her anxiety has taken over her life? Can that decline be reversed? Is it better to be Sally or Tricia? How much fear is enough? Can a person really change, or are Sally's present issues an inevitable and unchangeable product of her personality?

I hope to be able to answer some of these questions in this book. For now, let me just say this. Though many people suffering from anxiety disorders have been suffering for years, these conditions can all respond well to treatment. The reason that there are so many folks languishing with lives blighted by anxiety is that most people don't complain to their doctor about it. The withdrawal and avoidance that comes with these illnesses lies behind this, as does the shame which is their constant companion. So, if you know Sally or someone like her whose life is dominated by anxiety, the first step is to tell her *it isn't her fault*. She has an illness which makes her the way she is and which, up until now, has been out of her control. But it can be treated. Sally can escape the fear and misery that stalk her. She may have to push the system, as resources under the NHS are limited, but it's worth it as life can be better.

However, Sally (I know that isn't what you're called, but I never was any good at remembering names), I'm speaking to you now – if you are going to gain the relief from your symptoms which I hope for you, you'll need to promise me and yourself one thing from the start: that you'll try your hardest not to judge yourself and how well or badly you're doing at getting better. Treatment of anxiety disorders can be long, with ups and downs, advances and reverses, relapses and remissions. But over time, if you stick with it, things usually improve. You know what you're like though; you tend to blame yourself when anything goes wrong and to assume that any reverse means catastrophe will follow. You demand perfection from yourself and certainty of outcome from life. These aren't available here, so please just trust me for now. It isn't going to be as hard as you think, because *you don't need to fight your anxiety any more.* In fact, it's important that you don't; more on that later. Read this book and, when you're ready, go and see your GP. Tell her about your anxiety and ask to be referred for treatment. Then just put one foot in front of the other and see where treatment takes you. It'll be worth it. You may not believe it yet, but you are too.

Throughout this book, genders are alternated randomly when not referring to a specific gender. I have done this for ease and brevity of expression and it does not denote sex differences unless specified. Examples are given referring to one sex or the other to enable a real person to be visualized, but the gender of the examples was chosen at random and does not imply that the issues described are specific to or more predominant in either sex.

Part 1
ABOUT ANXIETY

1

What is anxiety and when is it an illness?

That's easy. Anxiety is fear. It's a normal, healthy emotion which nearly all of us experience (as I'll explain later, sociopaths don't get anxious). We need some anxiety, in the right place at the right time, in order to get ourselves going and to avoid too much danger. One of the reasons I kept somewhere near to schedule during my working life was because I was anxious to avoid my patients being cross with me for being kept waiting. Without anxiety, you would be unlikely to avoid that group of drunk football supporters milling around the railway station on a Saturday night. That would be a bad choice. A degree of anxiety helps us to make safe and well-judged decisions.

Anxiety is part of the 'fight-or-flight reaction'. We have inherited this response to perceived danger from our forebears and they from theirs, stretching right back to the lower primates, through natural selection. It's highly efficient, turning a resting animal into one that can run or fight to its maximum potential. That is achieved through the hormone adrenaline. This remarkable substance is released into the bloodstream automatically when the animal perceives threat. It worked really well when we lived on the primordial plain, making us pretty good at escaping from sabre-tooth tigers and the like. It causes an increase in heart rate, allowing more blood to be pumped around the body, targets blood to the muscles and internal organs where it is most needed in a crisis (you may notice that a person who is very anxious or shocked goes pale), causes sweating, allowing you to lose heat while running from or fighting with your pursuer, increases acuity of all the senses (things seem brighter, louder, sharper) and tends to encourage the bowels to empty from both ends (making you as light as possible enabling you to run as fast as you can, while also laying a confusing scent trail for the animal chasing you). Your muscles go into a state of tension, ready for a fight to the death, particularly the so-called 'ballistic' muscles in the arms, shoulders and legs, used for throwing, tearing, punching, kicking and running. Your shoulders tend to hunch up, making you the smallest possible target for a leaping animal or a thrown spear.

So anxiety works really well if you're being chased by a sabre-tooth tiger or someone with a very sharp weapon. Other specific forms of anxiety were equally adaptive in the distant past. For example, a fear of snakes or spiders probably increased our ancestors' chances of survival. Why is fear of snakes common, while fear of electricity is rare? The answer is that snakes and the danger some of them pose have been around for longer and so natural selection has had a chance to breed fear of them into

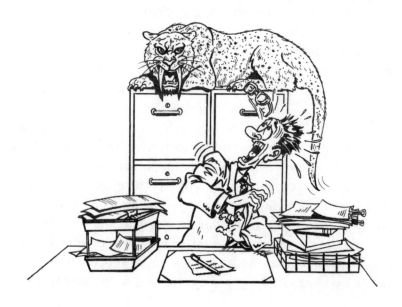

us. Fear of open spaces is, probably for good reason, common among small mammals. For example mice, which are low in the food chain, will always cross a room hugging the walls and, if prevented from doing so, will exhibit panic. So agoraphobia is adaptive, at least for rodents. However, there aren't that many situations or animals which threaten life and limb in most places where we live and work nowadays. Therein lies the problem. Our bodies are out of date, being designed for life as it was millions of years ago, not as it is now. Natural selection has stopped, as there aren't many things in our modern world which are likely to kill you before child-bearing age, which is what natural selection works on. And, in any case, our bodies don't know the difference between fear (anxiety) and anger (resentment). Either way, your body does the same thing, gets geared up for a fight to the death.

Anxiety is part of a continuum that extends from deep sleep, through relaxation, alertness, keyed-up, and on to terror and panic. The level at which you are able to function depends on your level of arousal. As you will see from Figure 1 (called the Yerkes–Dodson curve after the researchers who first drew it), there is a fairly broad plateau of arousal at which you're able to function at your peak, but the fall-off when it happens is sudden and precipitous. It only takes a little more arousal to go from being on top of your game to dissembling in panic.

The problems occur when your arousal level or the degree of fear you experience is out of kilter with the situation you find yourself in. Or if you are fearful all of the time. Or if fear is automatically generated by specific harmless objects or situations. Or if the fear you suffer stops you from acting as you would or doing the things you would choose to do, were it at the level experienced by most other people. Or if your fear generates feelings, sensations or symptoms which cause you to suffer (and which increase your fear, leading to a vicious cycle). Or if you keep falling over the edge of the Yerkes–Dodson curve.

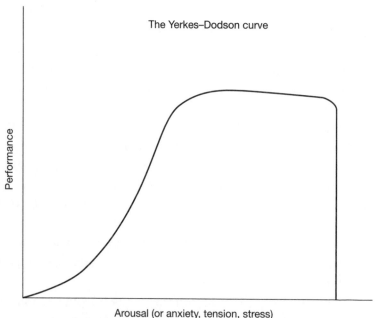

Figure 1 The Yerkes–Dodson curve

Or if the real reason why you're so wound up is that you're angry and resentful.

If your fear is disabling, not just for a moment but repeatedly or constantly, you have an illness, an anxiety disorder. If you do, you're not alone, though it may feel as if you are. In fact, anxiety disorders are very common. Nearly one in three women and one in five men will suffer from one or other of these conditions at some point in their lives. About one in ten suffer panic attacks, at least occasionally, and a similar number have specific phobias (such as animals, contamination etc.). One in seven suffer with social phobia (social anxiety disorder) and one in thirty suffer with agoraphobia. Between one in ten and one in twenty are disabled by constant anxiety (that is, fear without a specific focus). Up to one in twenty of the population are disabled by health anxiety and this rises to one in five people sitting in a

GP waiting room. Anxiety disorders are common, especially in women, who are afflicted roughly twice as often as men. People who are separated, divorced, unemployed or a home-maker (housewife or househusband) are at greater risk of suffering from an anxiety disorder, as are those who for any reason are isolated from the social supports that sustain most of us.

There is a big overlap between anxiety disorders and depressive illness (major depression). Most people suffering with a depressive illness are also plagued by anxiety. While the majority of those suffering with anxiety disorders don't have a depressive illness, most are prone to low mood, sometimes severely so. If the worst aspect of your suffering is deep, black depression, I would suggest you read one of my other books, *Depressive Illness: The curse of the strong* and, please, go to see your GP.

Anxiety comes in lots of different shapes and sizes. I've mentioned most of the different types of anxiety disorders already, but it's worth describing them in a bit more detail. Just one aside: I'm not going to deal with obsessive-compulsive disorder (OCD) in this book. While it is a condition driven by anxiety, it is a very big subject and deserves its own book. The same is true for post-traumatic stress disorder (PTSD). Fortunately, there are several excellent books available to help people who suffer from those conditions.

Generalized anxiety disorder (GAD) is a state of constant fearfulness, a sense that disaster is waiting around the corner, ready to pounce once your back is turned. This is often at the core of the condition; a feeling that you have to be constantly alert to danger, lest it catch you unawares. You are constantly worrying, however hard you try not to. You vigilantly scan your environment, searching for signs that something is wrong. Your muscles are always tense and, because they are ballistic not postural muscles, they aren't designed to be in tension for long periods and so tend to cramp up. Your pulse rate, breathing and

7

blood pressure tend to be on the high side and you tend towards loose bowels and a 'churning stomach'. In other words, you are more or less constantly under the effects of adrenaline. You tend to have difficulty sleeping, you can't relax and you are often jumpy and irritable. That is, your brain is in a state of constant overarousal, running too hot all the time.

Someone suffering from panic disorder (PD) on the other hand tends to be less anxious for much of the time. Either out of the blue, or triggered by specific circumstances, a full-blown fight-or-flight reaction occurs (a panic attack) with breathlessness, racing heartbeat, sweating, nausea, an urge to escape and sometimes a feeling that you are going to faint or even die (you won't). If the panic attacks are linked to social phobia, you may experience blushing. While some people have both generalized anxiety and panic attacks, some really aren't exceptionally anxious between attacks. You may even wake up at night with a panic attack.

Phobic anxiety disorder (PAD) is a catch-all label, referring to anxiety generated by specific objects (such as certain animals) or situations (such as being trapped in enclosed spaces). Fear grows as you anticipate the situation, producing the symptoms of anxiety which I have outlined, leading to avoidance and, over time, to an increase in the fear you experience, which can only be allayed by further avoidance. And so it goes on.

I find it useful to separate out two types of phobia, as they have a lot of aspects that are different from the types of PAD I have described, and they are agoraphobia and social anxiety disorder (SAD).

Agoraphobia (AP) is literally a fear of open spaces. In practice, it usually means you become increasingly fearful the further you are from home or the environment where you feel safe and secure. As you leave your safe place, you suffer increasingly severe anxiety and the physical symptoms which go with it. You may suffer panic attacks and the *fear of fear* spiral causes you to be as fearful of the attacks as of the situation itself. As you will gather, there is a big overlap between agoraphobia and PD. You fear that you will lose control, causing you to embarrass yourself in public, or that you will faint, die or go mad (you won't).

Social anxiety disorder (also called social phobia (SP)) is an often quite disabling condition resulting from an excessive sensitivity to the opinions of others, in turn usually caused by low self-esteem and shyness. In social situations you feel inadequate and exposed and you are overwhelmed by a fear of embarrassing yourself. Commonly, you fear blushing and you imagine that everyone will see your face flush and judge you for it. The anxiety this causes may lead to some blushing, confirming your fears. You may fear losing control of your bowels and again this fear may lead to some urgency in needing the toilet, or you may fear your body shaking, leading to a tremor in your hands. SP may be restricted to situations in which you have to perform, such as public speaking, or may involve any situation in which you have to interact with people.

Health anxiety disorder (HAD) refers to a condition in which you are constantly preoccupied by a fear of serious (or fatal) illness. You may or may not have a diagnosed physical illness, but the point is that the severity of your anxiety and the degree of suffering which your symptoms cause you is out of proportion to the underlying physical pathology in your body. There's the problem. How do you know that there isn't something major and potentially fatal lying behind the symptoms you are experiencing? Maybe your doctor just hasn't found it yet. The truth is that you can never be 100 per cent certain about anything, but most doctors accept that there is a limit to how many investigations should be carried out when each one before has failed to find something that needs treatment. If you suffer with HAD you can't stop looking for a cause of your discomfort, being sure that something catastrophic underlies it. You spend every minute of every day ruminating anxiously about your fears and, as we've discussed, that anxiety causes more symptoms. When I explain this, you answer angrily: 'So you're saying it's all in my head are you?' No, I'm not. Your symptoms and the suffering they cause you are real. The only questions are what causes them and how can they best be treated? This is, in my view, the most difficult type of anxiety disorder to treat. The dividing line between your doctor listening to and respecting your concerns and following up on them on the one hand, and making things worse by over-investigation on the other is blurred. I think I have an answer to this conundrum, but more on that later.

So who gets these conditions? I'm going to deal with what causes them and how they develop in the next chapter, but for now I will just observe that most of those who came to see me suffering with anxiety disorders were people who had a very low opinion of themselves (and the world and the future). They were ashamed of themselves. Now, there are people in the world who really should be ashamed of themselves (think Palace of Westminster, The White House, Kremlin), but not these folks, who *try so hard*. Those who should be aren't, but those who shouldn't be are. Hmm, maybe there's a key there ...

From here on, I will use the following abbreviations for brevity:

Generalized anxiety disorder – GAD   *Phobic anxiety disorder* – PAD
Panic disorder – PD   *Agoraphobia* – AP
Social anxiety disorder – SAD   *Health anxiety disorder* – HAD

2

What causes anxiety disorders?

When, in the 1950s, British Prime Minister Harold Macmillan was asked by a journalist what in political life he most feared, he replied: 'Events, dear boy, events.' So the story goes. Or as Americans like to say: 'S—t happens.' So is that it? Is it the stuff which happens to us which makes us anxious? Do people believe that life is going to keep going wrong the way it has up until now? Are the most anxious people those who have endured the most adversity? Well, to an extent, but there's a lot more to it than that. It looks as though the loss of hope that things will get better has more to do with depression than anxiety. If depression is despairing of anything improving, of mourning what has been lost, then anxiety is fear that things will get worse, that what you have will be taken away. As such, it has always seemed to me that in seeking to deal with disabling anxiety we need to look at our relationship with the future more than the past.

Genes

But to do that we have to understand where anxiety comes from, so let's start at the beginning, with our genes. It does look as though our tendency to anxiety is, to a large extent, passed down from our parents. A part of that effect is genetic; this has been established by studies looking at the chances of a non-identical twin suffering with anxiety if their twin has an anxiety disorder, and comparing these with identical twins where one has the condition. This separates out the effect of genes (the same in identical twins but different in non-identical twins) and environmental/learning factors (the same in both). Unfortunately, the research isn't completely clear on this question, but it looks like what you learn in childhood is more important than the genes you carry, at least for most types of anxiety disorder. With GAD, there may be a bigger genetic influence, but this may be because of the common ground between GAD and depressive illness (depression has a strong genetic component), which I mentioned in Chapter 1.

In summary, blaming your anxiety on your genes doesn't work.

Brain physiology and chemistry

Biological psychiatrists have been trying to explain anxiety disorders in terms of abnormal functioning of one or another brain part or system for years without, as yet, consistent success. The number of theories abound and, frankly, it makes my head spin, but a few things are clear and worth understanding.

Fear seems to be generated mainly in a structure deep within the brain called the amygdala. This structure is programmed to discharge impulses to other parts of the brain in response to perceived threat, or even lack of evidence of safety. The effect is to switch these structures on, in particular those in the brain stem and another structure, the hypothalamus, which together control the fight-or-flight reaction and the body's longer-term responses to stress. The amygdala is a primitive structure, which we have in common with all primates, and it acts automatically, unless it is prevented from doing so. The only supervision the amygdala has is from the cerebral cortex: the conscious, 'thinking' part of the brain. That is, unless we consciously control our fear, it controls us, careering around like a rudderless ship in a storm with the amygdala at its centre.

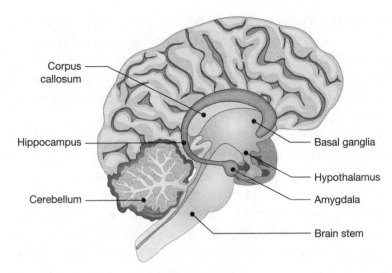

Figure 2 The amygdala, cortex and brain stem

When the amygdala is active it triggers a cascade of events, the result of which is, in the short term, a release of adrenaline, thus setting up the fight-or-flight reaction. In the longer term though, if the danger it faces persists, the body has different priorities, needing to slow things down to encourage the animal to withdraw from danger and to reduce inflammation. This is achieved through the hypothalamus triggering a series of events which culminate in the release of the hormone cortisol. This is a hormone which slows down metabolism and inflammatory processes. The body is smart that way: in the short term, it releases adrenaline to maximize the chance of winning a fight or successfully escaping it; in the longer term, if the danger remains, it releases cortisol which maximizes the chance of staying out of danger and allowing healing to occur. Thus, adrenaline is the short-term stress hormone and cortisol the long-term stress hormone.

A baby is an unprogrammed computer. Childhood is about the brain getting programmed and calibrating its settings. If a child suffers a lot of stress, fear or trauma early in life, her amygdala and hypothalamus become primed for danger; that is, the dial gets turned up. As the child reaches adulthood, she is then primed to respond to situations as stresses, triggering the stress responses which the brain has available. She is super-sensitive both to external cues suggesting danger and to internal ones.

One of these is the blood carbon dioxide (CO_2) level. High levels of CO_2 (suggesting suffocation) cause the amygdala to switch on and fear to be generated in everyone. However, in those whose amygdala has been made super-sensitive through early life stress, *low* levels of CO_2 (resulting from increased breathing rate) will also switch on the amygdala. So someone who has been sensitized to stress as a child will have anxiety switched on if they get *too much* air into their lungs. Such a person faces a double whammy – a super-sensitive amygdala ready to switch on the stress response, including breathlessness, at the drop of a hat, and a trigger which responds to the increased intake or air by ratcheting up the body's stress response still further. For most of us, our body reacts to danger. For someone primed to be anxious, she reacts to her body. That is, if her body shows signs of stress, she presumes danger exists. Vicious cycles of spiralling anxiety are the result.

In terms of the chemicals that are active in the brain, three transmitter chemicals (substances which allow the transmission of nerve impulses from one nerve to the next) appear to be involved. Noradrenaline seems to be overactive, GABA (gamma-aminobutyric acid) underactive and serotonin either overactive or underactive. Confused? So am I. It only matters because medicines used to treat anxiety work on these systems. The opiate system is also involved, which is why drugs such as morphine and heroin cause sedation and lowered anxiety (though they cause increased anxiety if taken regularly). We actually produce our own opiate-like substances called endorphins, which give us a feeling of calm wellbeing and they don't come with the problems posed by opiate drugs. Certain habits, such as exercise and meditation, stimulate the endorphin system.

Take-away message: if you've suffered from anxiety all your life, it isn't a weakness of character or all in your mind. There is a problem with your brain's programming and settings. They can be fixed, but that will require a change in the way you think and your habits.

Personality

I have often had people say to me: 'I've always been anxious, it's just my personality.' The implication is that nothing can change because personality is fixed.

But it isn't. Personality changes all the time. I'm a very different person now from the one I was at the age of 20 and, when I was working, I was very different at work from how I was at home. Like everyone, my personality changed to fit my circumstances. What is personality anyway? I think it is best defined by the product of your behaviours. If you say that someone is 'outgoing', you mean that they go out and socialize a lot. If you call them 'confident', you mean they act confidently. Who knows how they feel inside? Actually, if they have been behaving confidently for a long time, they probably do feel confident now, because of the basic psychological principle that *you become the way that you act*. It's why so many kids got into difficulty playing with Ouija boards back in the 1970s. It wasn't that they were getting possessed by the spirits they were communing with, but just that if you behave bizarrely for long enough, you become bizarre. It's also why that excellent organization Alcoholics Anonymous (AA) tells their members to 'fake it to make it'. Go through the motions and you'll get that way in the end.

Here is the problem that I have with many researchers in this field who talk of 'vulnerability factors' lying behind both anxiety and depression. Yes, people suffering with anxiety disorders sometimes are sensitive and introspective, with a low opinion of themselves at the same time as having excessively high expectations of themselves. But these traits can also be seen as strengths. Most of the good people who do the best and most selfless things have these traits. The question isn't how to eradicate these traits in your makeup, but how to stop them leading to you becoming ill. As with anything, extremes can be a problem, so people with extremes in their makeup (sometimes called personality disorders) do sometimes suffer with long-term anxiety, but these form only a small minority of those with anxiety disorders and I won't deal with their issues here.

So when dealing with anxiety disorders, yes, some people have struggled with fear for most of their lives, but I don't think that using 'personality' as an explanation is particularly helpful.

Learning

Back to the computer with which a baby is born and which needs to be programmed. A child does this by learning from her environment. The main ways in which this is achieved are through didactic teaching, vicarious learning, and classical and operant conditioning.

Didactic teaching means a parent, teacher or peer telling or showing the child about the world and how they can best interact with it. An example would be 'Don't accept sweets from strangers, because not all of them are as nice as they seem to be'. A child needs to be taught an appropriate degree of anxiety to be safe.

Vicarious learning refers to the process of learning achieved by watching what does and doesn't work for others. Seeing your friend falling off his bicycle and grazing his knee because of riding too fast around a corner would be an example.

Classical conditioning is the process of learning a response from repetitive pairing of stimuli. Pavlov trained his dogs to salivate to the sound of a buzzer and other stimuli by pairing the stimulus with giving the dog food to eat many times over. Eventually the dog salivates in response to the buzzer or stimulus alone, even when no food is present, though if you keep sounding the buzzer without producing food, eventually the dog will stop salivating at the sound of the buzzer (*extinction*). If a child is scratched more than once by the family's tabby, he may develop a fear of cats. This depends on him avoiding cats, because if he approaches cats several times and is able to stroke them without getting scratched, extinction occurs. However, each time the child gets scratched, his fear increases, it is *reinforced*.

Operant conditioning refers to the process of learning from the results of your own actions. If a rat is rewarded with food each time it presses a bar in its cage, it will eventually press the bar regularly whether or not food is presented. Again, extinction will occur eventually if the action is not rewarded. To an extent, punishment has the opposite effect, so if pressing the bar causes an electric shock to be administered, the rat will, not surprisingly, learn to avoid the bar. In practice, punishment seems not to be as effective as reward. If the shock is too severe, the rat is so traumatized by the experience that it fails to learn from it. In humans, things are a bit more complicated owing to our more complex emotions. What is a reward? Is it a gift, food, a pat on the back, a kind word, or even being allowed to avoid the thing you've learnt to be afraid of? However illogical your fear may be, avoiding the object or situation which generates it is very rewarding (this is called *negative reinforcement*).

The thing is that most people with phobias don't have a clear history of trauma related to the object of their phobia. Most people with a fear of heights have never been injured in a fall, and most people who have suffered such an injury don't develop any phobia. Here's where thinking comes in. You don't actually have to experience an injury from falling to become fearful of heights. Just imagining it can make you frightened and the experience of your physical reaction to this fear may be sufficient trauma in itself to increase your fear further, leading you to avoid heights altogether. Each time you are asked to climb a ladder you become fearful, which is unpleasant, but each time you refuse, you experience relief of this fear, which is reinforcing. Extinction never happens because, regardless of the fact that you have never fallen, your fear and its release when you avoid heights keeps it going.

In any case, learning can sometimes occur even when you're not aware that it's happening. A child may not be aware of the fact that mum tends to be irritable on Fridays, at the end of a long week with no support at home, that he fears mum's tempers or that fish is always served on Fridays (being a Catholic family). Nonetheless, the child develops a fear of eating fish.

A further subtlety is that people, as opposed to animals, are more aware of context. A dog may be trained to respond in a certain way every time you clap your hands, while a human knows the difference between a clap of the hands delivered with an icy stare and one given with a warm smile. It's therefore much more difficult to know how people will react to conditioning than it is with animals.

I think that the most important form of learning in this context is *learned helplessness.*

Returning to the rat in the cage pressing a bar. What if you sometimes give it food when it presses the bar, but sometimes give it an electric shock instead? Or you sometimes give it food and sometimes not? Or sometimes it has to press the bar once a minute to avoid a shock, but sometimes it has to be once a second. There are no consistent rules and the rat learns only one thing: it doesn't matter what I do, it won't make any difference in the end. I have no control over what happens. I'm powerless.

If you then let the rat out of the cage and let a fierce and hungry cat into the room, the rat will behave strangely. It sits in the middle of the floor, apparently paralysed by fear, and lets itself be eaten.

The rat has learnt to be helpless, that bad things will happen and that it is powerless to prevent them. Torturers in dictatorships are taught this principle in their basic training. Don't always beat your victim, sometimes be nice to him. Keep him guessing. Teach him that he has no influence over what happens to him. That way, he loses his will and knows only powerlessness and fear.

A child needs to learn that the world is predictable and controllable. That what she does makes a difference. If she doesn't, she will learn to be helpless and fearful. You don't have to be cruel for this to happen, just to be inconsistent and unpredictable. Who said parenting was easy?

The result of poor learning experiences in life, particularly early on, is to cause you to develop a distorted view of things. The psychologist Aaron Beck described a 'negative cognitive triad' in people who go on to develop major depression but, in fact, those suffering from anxiety disorders often have the same distorted perspective on things. The triad is a negative view of *yourself, the world and the future*. If you start from a basis of expecting the worst, you're both going to fear a great many things and to tend to avoid them. You will tend to expect the worst thing that your imagination can construct. You will catastrophize.

Psychoanalysts see anxiety as being generated by psychological conflicts, mostly picked up early in childhood. I'm not going to go into these theories here, as the advice I have on how to manage anxiety disorders doesn't rely on them. It doesn't mean they aren't relevant, just that they aren't what this book is about. I will say this though: conflicting needs are stressful. If you have a demanding job, that is anxiety-provoking enough. So is having a lot of domestic and family responsibilities. If you have both, there aren't enough hours in the day or energy in your body to do everything. Your needs are in conflict and these conflicting demands increase the stress on you not by a factor of two, but of ten. Ever wondered why women, who in the modern world still shoulder more than their fair share of domestic and family responsibilities, suffer from anxiety disorders more commonly than men?

Cognitive dissonance

This is defined as the distance between your ideal self and your real self. If your ideal is perfection and, particularly, if you feel you should achieve your ideal, you are condemning yourself to repeated frustration and failure. Any enterprise you take on will inevitably be accompanied by fear, as you know that you can't succeed and that you will react to your failure with vicious self-criticism. The little guy in the cartoon below, who appears in most of my books, is pumping weights because his ideal self is a superhuman man-mountain. He'll never

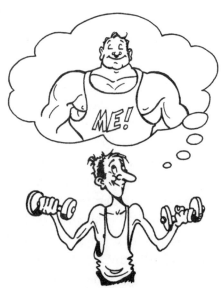

Cognitive dissonance

succeed as his body isn't made that way and he feels anxious in social situations, as he feels people will judge his physical appearance. He ignores his many fine qualities and talents and only seeks what he can't have, the appearance of an international rugby player.

Researchers have found that reducing cognitive dissonance by developing more realistic and achievable goals and an accurate self-image is a central characteristic of all effective psychological therapies.

Life events and resonance

It would be great if adversity made you stronger but, in my experience, it doesn't; it makes you more vulnerable, particularly to future adversity of the same kind. The earlier in life the adversity happens, the more profound and enduring are its effects. People who have had mainly negative experiences in childhood tend to expect the worst from the future. They fear what they have experienced before, really or symbolically.

Susan's father was unpredictable, often loving but also prone to bouts of temper. He sadly died suddenly and unexpectedly of a heart attack when Susan was aged 12. Everyone was impressed by her resilience and how much of a support she managed to be to her mother in the months that followed, even though her mum had difficulty coping with her grief and had little love or warmth to give to her kids, who were largely left to look after themselves. Susan became very protective of her younger siblings and worked even harder at school than she had before. She was a rock. Twenty years later, Susan is doing well in her career, but there are rumours of redundancies in the offing. Her mother, who had helped her with childcare, has a fall and injures her leg, meaning that Susan has to try to find another solution at short notice. She becomes increasingly anxious, both at work and at home, leading to a reduction in her level of performance in her job and strains in her relationship with her husband.

What is happening here? Losing your father isn't the same as the threat of losing your job, or unexpectedly losing your childcare, are they? Well no, not literally, but symbolically they are. All involve a disappearance of certainty and of a sense that bad things and loss won't happen. Susan expects to lose her job and is paralysed by fear because loss is what she experienced in her formative years. This fear manifests as irritability at home and the resulting tension reduces the support she receives, ratcheting the pressure up further. Had she enjoyed a childhood without major loss and with uninterrupted predictability, boundaries and love, she would have been able to absorb much better the difficulties and threats she now faces. This way in which adverse experiences, especially early in life, magnify the effect of symbolically similar effects later on is caused 'resonance'. If you experience more fear in a situation than it merits, this may be because of resonance with past events.

Changes in the world

That life is more complicated than it used to be is a truism. It's not that it's more or less stressful, just that the stresses we face have changed. And that's the point, change is a stress. This is a point which business leaders and politicians either don't get or wilfully ignore. Leaders tend to be like dogs. When you introduce your mutt to a new garden, he has to go and urinate around the perimeter, to lay a marker showing that it's his territory. Leaders increasingly seem to need to do the same. When a new one comes into post he inevitably changes everything, presumably to show that the business/district/country or whatever is *his*. In my experience men are worse in this regard than women (I realize that's a generalization, but it's just my opinion). Unfortunately, this puts a much greater load on everyone. The casual cynics find a way around the system, seeming to comply when in fact changing very little; while the honest, diligent triers attempt to carry out their leader's edicts to the letter, getting increasingly stressed along the way and, as often as not, appearing in my office with an anxiety disorder.

It's not that change can be avoided; any business which doesn't change with the times will go under. But it should be introduced carefully, recognizing the harm it can do if imposed without thought.

One of the biggest changes in recent years has been in technology. Old buffers like me tend to resist much of this (you won't find me on Facebook or Twitter), but younger people can't. It's how life is led nowadays. The generation that has grown up never knowing a time when iPhone, Android and similar devices didn't exist has been called 'iGen'. They do seem to be suffering from more anxiety disorders than the generation before them and much of this appears to be attributable to social media. There is immense pressure to get 'likes' on your Facebook page and cyber bullying is easier than pushing someone around in the playground. In one study, a group of iGens were split into two groups, one of which stopped using social media for three months while the other continued as normal. The group who went without Facebook and the like became significantly less anxious and depressed, only to sink back to the state of their media-connected peers within weeks of resuming their smartphone use. Other researchers have looked at the effect of limiting time spent online and using social media, finding equally compelling results.

What makes anxiety worse?

Once anxiety has started, it tends to feed on itself. Being anxious, and particularly the physical symptoms of anxiety, is scary and unpleasant, setting up a spiral of *fear of fear*. This is most marked in panic attacks. Anyone who has suffered one will know that panic attacks are horrid. But many other factors serve to perpetuate and exacerbate anxiety which is already present.

Avoidance is a natural response to what frightens us, but it is also the fuel on which anxiety feeds. If you get bitten by a dog, all you need to develop a phobia of dogs is to avoid them for a while. The longer you avoid them, the worse the phobia gets. And avoiding things can cause some of the problems you fear in any case. Say you fear having a heart attack. Your anxiety causes breathlessness and sometimes crampy pains in your chest (from tension in your chest muscles). You avoid exercise because it tends to bring on these sensations, which make you feel as if you're having a heart attack. As a result, your weight increases and your risk of developing cardiovascular disease increases.

So avoidance is to be avoided, when possible. This change is probably best done gradually (systematic desensitization, see Chapter 7) if you have severe anxiety, particularly if it relates to something specific, but if something makes you only a bit anxious and you are able to approach the object or situation without too much distress, do so. For example, if you tend not to like driving on busy motorways because you once had a minor accident on one, try not to avoid motorways altogether. Use them occasionally, when it makes sense to do so.

Alcohol is the tranquillizing drug that we use more than any other. The trouble is that it's a very bad drug. An effective pharmaceutical product has the desired effect, few and only minor side effects, has a broad range of safe and effective dosages, and has little or no tolerance (meaning that it doesn't lose its efficacy over time when taken regularly). Alcohol fails these tests spectacularly. Yes, it reduces anxiety in some situations, but not reliably. We all know what happens if you drink too much and it isn't pretty. Taken regularly to excess it harms more or less every organ and system in the body (I won't expand on this here, but if you want more information, go to my book on the subject: *Dying for a Drink*).

Most importantly in the context of anxiety, alcohol not only loses its efficacy over time, it actually makes anxiety worse in the long term. Much worse. Figure 3 illustrates this. Each time you take a drink your anxiety reduces, but what you don't notice is that when the effect wears off, your level of anxiety goes back up, not to where it was before you started drinking, but slightly higher. This increase is sufficiently small each time you drink not to be noticeable but, over time, if you drink heavily every day your anxiety level will ratchet up steadily. 'Oh, but alcohol is the only thing which calms me down,' you say. Well yes, it does in the short term, but the opposite happens in the long term. 'That can't be right,' you say, 'because last time I stopped drinking I felt much more anxious.' Yes, you did, because you were suffering from the withdrawal effects of alcohol, one of which is increased anxiety. This is only short term though, as you can see from Figure 3. If you stay off the booze for more than a week or two, your anxiety level will eventually fall back to where it was before you started drinking. I'll come back to this, but don't try to stop drinking abruptly without medical help if you are severely dependent on alcohol. Conversely, drinking moderately, up to two or three units a day (a pint of beer or two small glasses of wine) and not every day is very unlikely to lead to problems.

Some other drugs that reduce anxiety come with similar problems to alcohol, although booze is one of the worst. Taking tranquillizers such as diazepam (Valium) or lorazepam (Ativan) doesn't tend to work well in the long term. Their efficacy gradually falls over time and, if they are stopped abruptly after long-term use, a rebound increase in anxiety can occur. Short-term use is OK but, if you've had severe anxiety for a long time, a brief course of tranquillizers isn't going to solve anything. Other stronger drugs, with worse addictive

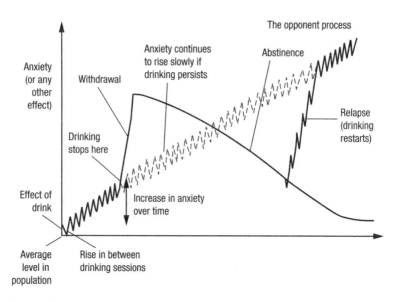

Figure 3 The opponent process

potential, include opiates such as morphine and heroin, illicit tranquillizers such as ketamine and older tranquillizers such as barbiturates and chlormethiazole (Heminevrin). I'm not too sure about cannabis. It doesn't seem to have the problems I've described above to any great degree, but its effect isn't reliable. I have seen people suffering from a dramatic worsening of their anxiety after taking pot. Strangely, some people suffering from anxiety take stimulants such as amphetamines or cocaine, believing that they need a 'high' to increase their confidence. Stimulants make anxiety worse.

The one set of drugs that stand apart are the 'SSRIs', a class of antidepressants which appear to have sustained efficacy against anxiety (after the first two weeks, during which anxiety sometimes increases), at least for some. Problems usually occur only if you allow these drugs to be your *only* solution to your anxiety. More on this later.

Reassurance can be addictive. It's not harmful in itself; occasionally it can help you to face your fears, but dependence on reassurance produces some of the same problems as dependence on drugs. The more you get the more you need. The trouble is that it tends to disappear suddenly, leading to rebound increase in anxiety akin to a drug withdrawal effect. Mike suffers from HAD. His friend Ed is a nurse and regularly reassures Mike that his symptoms are unlikely to represent serious physical pathology. Mike finds Ed's reassurance very comforting, but he starts to need it more and more often. He ends up phoning Ed several times a day. Ed does his best to be a good friend but, over time, he becomes exhausted and resentful of the demands Mike puts upon him and, one day, he suddenly withdraws his support, leaving Mike with no way of seeing things realistically or keeping his fears in check.

Like everything else, reassurance has to be used sparingly and judiciously if it isn't going to make things worse.

3

Anxiety as a symptom and a cause

In addition to the anxiety disorders outlined in Chapter 1, anxiety is a symptom present in many illnesses, both physical and mental. For this reason, a sudden, unexpected and unexplained increase in your level of anxiety is worth a visit to your GP. Having said this, there are many more cases of people whose health-related anxiety has no physical basis than there are of those whose anxiety is caused by physical illness. If your doctor is confident that there is no major physical pathology underlying your symptoms, your best hope of escaping your symptoms will be to pursue psychological therapy, of which more later. However, it is important to be aware of anxiety as a symptom of other conditions, as treating the anxiety can often improve your response to the other treatments you receive for your condition.

Physical conditions

It can be quite difficult for you to distinguish between the physical effects of anxiety and of physical conditions. For example, palpitations, increased heart rate and a feeling of fear may occur if you have an overactive thyroid gland or, less commonly, an overactive adrenal gland. Many people suffering with atrial fibrillation are unaware that their heartbeat is irregular, although they may experience palpitations similar to when they are anxious. Breathlessness is a symptom of anxiety and panic, but also of respiratory and cardiac diseases. Numbness or tingling in the hands or feet may reflect anxiety or, less commonly, neurological disease. Abdominal discomfort and bloating can occur as a symptom of anxiety disorders or of a number of bowel conditions. The point here is that, while it may be impossible for you to determine the origin of your symptoms, it isn't usually difficult for your doctor to distinguish between symptoms caused by anxiety or by underlying physical disease. If she then recommends psychological treatment, it doesn't mean that she is dismissing your symptoms or labelling them as 'all in your head'. For example, there is good evidence that reducing anxiety in patients with established heart disease significantly improves their outcomes.

Mental illnesses

As I have explained, there is no real division between mind and body, so it would be fair to criticize me for making a false distinction in separating physical and mental illnesses. However, they are conventionally labelled separately, which is why I've put them in different sections here.

Nearly everyone suffering from major depression (depressive illness, clinical depression) also suffers with anxiety. Is anxiety merely a symptom, or is it a central driver of the illness? Do antidepressants work for major depression mainly by reducing anxiety? I don't know the answers to these questions, but what has been clear to me over the years I've treated depressed patients is that reducing their levels of anxiety is an important part of treatment. Some don't look anxious, such as those suffering so-called 'retarded depression' (where depression leads to almost total withdrawal and inactivity), but that is only because their extreme lack of energy and motivation doesn't allow them to give expression to the fear they are experiencing. Once they recover, these patients tell me that overwhelming fear was mixed in with despair and hopelessness in equal measure when they were ill.

People suffering from bipolar affective disorder (formerly known as manic depressive illness) suffer enormous fluctuations of mood from extreme elation to deep depression, each phase lasting sometimes several weeks. Not surprisingly, in the depressed phase sufferers are tormented by anxiety, but even in the high phase anxiety may be a feature. The elevated mood is sometimes accompanied by agitation, restlessness, irritability, insomnia and, particularly in the transition from mania to depression, fear.

In psychotic illnesses such as schizophrenia, anxiety is again a prominent symptom. Indeed, it seems that sufferers from these debilitating illnesses are among the most anxious people in existence. Some suffer from persecutory delusions which further ramp up their fear. Reducing anxiety levels is again crucial to successful treatment.

People suffering from extremes of personality development (sometimes called personality disorder) are often plagued by anxiety. One such category, 'borderline personality disorder', is characterized by intense and unstable emotions, instability of relationships, repeated crises, a feeling of emptiness and a tendency to explosive outbursts or self-harming behaviours. Not surprisingly, a large part of the suffering these individuals experience is driven by anxiety.

Anxiety as a cause of illness

Anxiety, as I've discussed, is a normal adaptive emotion. But too much of it for too long is toxic. Long-term severe anxiety causes a whole range of bodily changes, none of which are good. In particular, blood pressure goes up, blood sugar is raised, fats are released by the liver into the blood stream, stomach acid levels rise and bowels become increasingly active and, eventually, inflamed. As explained in Chapter 1, hormonal changes occur which increase these effects. In addition, behaviours developed in response to anxiety, such as withdrawal, lack of exercise and excessive consumption of food and alcohol, also serve to exacerbate these changes. So, as you can see, long-term severe anxiety is a major contributor to heart disease, stroke risk, type 2 diabetes, stomach ulcers and bowel disorders, including irritable bowel syndrome (IBS). Likewise, inflammatory conditions such as Crohn's disease and rheumatoid arthritis are sensitive to raised anxiety levels. Equally, suffering from such conditions is very anxiety-provoking, so there is a vicious cycle at play.

The set of conditions sometimes called 'Medically Unexplained' sit in an area where anxiety is both a symptom and part of the cause. Diseases such as chronic fatigue syndrome (myalgic encephalomyelitis (ME)), fibromyalgia and IBS are real physical illnesses, but then so is major depression. Anxiety plays a major role both in driving these illnesses and as a symptom of them, just as is the case with the other illnesses listed here. I'll say it again: *there is no division between mind and body, mental and physical.* Nothing is imaginary, your suffering is real, but that doesn't mean that your anxiety is unimportant or that reducing it doesn't matter.

You may wonder why I'm telling you all this, as the object is to make you less, not more anxious. The point I'm keen to get across though is that everything is linked. If everything medical is being done to treat your physical illness, or if your doctor has done everything reasonable to find the origin of your symptoms, there is still something else that can be done. That something is reducing your level of anxiety.

4

People who aren't anxious

You can learn something from anyone. Everyone, even the person you like or respect least, has something you can learn from. You just have to notice. So, if you have too much anxiety, if you fear too much, it's worth looking first at those who have little or no fear and, second, at those who do but are able to control it really well.

In the former group, those with no anxiety at all, are the *sociopaths* (psychopaths). These folks have little in the way of feelings of any kind, not by choice, but because they just don't *feel*. This usually results from a combination of genetics, brutal experiences and a lack of any consistent instruction on morality (or anything else) in childhood. They have no conscience, no empathy, no anxiety and no appreciation of right and wrong. There is only opportunity and impulse. Sociopaths can't learn from their mistakes, because to do so you need access to feelings of guilt, regret or remorse, and the ability to equate your action to its consequence. Operant conditioning (see Chapter 2) doesn't operate in a sociopath. If sociopath Jack punches Bill in the face, there is no point in telling him he shouldn't have done it or that it was wrong, or in pointing out the pain and suffering he has caused Bill. He will be perplexed and reply something like: 'Why are you getting at me? Bill was in my way and that was inconvenient. I wanted to hit him, so I did.' You can punish him all you like, send him to jail if you so choose, but I can guarantee that once he's out, the next time someone gets in his way the same thing will happen. You would think that sociopaths, with their lack of fear, would be good soldiers, but I'm told that the army is quite careful to exclude them, because Jack is just as likely to shoot his commanding officer as he is the enemy.

What can we learn from Jack? He is at the end of a spectrum, with him at one end and someone suffering from severe GAD at the other. We don't want to be like Jack; he's really disabled, unable to function effectively in a society demanding adherence to social mores and an engagement with rules of give and take. What we need is to move to the centre ground, where we have some fear, but not too much or in the wrong situations and not all the time. The feeling and your response to it needs to fit the situation. You need to have some control over your emotions.

I've treated a number of soldiers in my time. Almost all had been effective warriors, most had faced danger with heroism and several had won medals for bravery. In fact, it seemed that the braver the soldier, the more likely he was eventually to need treatment from someone like me. These men and women didn't lack fear, but they had learnt how to control it when in the heat of battle. The fact that they had done so with such success meant that they experienced more than their fair share of trauma, from which they were affected as much as the next person. Their bravery resulted from an ability, temporarily, to put their fear to one side in order to do what needed to be done, that is to exercise choice rather than to be controlled by their fear. They dealt with the foe in front of them, rather than thinking forward to the possible injury or death which might result from their actions. For one reason or another, they had gained the ability to stay present when it mattered.

Turning to less weighty subjects, I've got pretty good at predicting who will succeed in major sporting events such as golf or tennis majors and international cricket fixtures. It isn't always the most skilful players. What is needed when coming in to bat at 20 for 3 in an Ashes Test or having a one-shot lead in the final round of the Open, is not a will to win. We all want to win, some of us so much that we get paralysed by anxiety that we might fail to do so. No, the major winners are those who are able to accept that they will sometimes fail and so are able to give it their best, ball by ball, shot by shot, without thinking forward to the result. After losing a Wimbledon final he was expected to win, Boris Becker was asked if he was devastated. 'No,' he replied, 'I gave it my best and it didn't go my way today. I'll probably win next year.' He did.

Next, let's look at a hotchpotch of careless, selfish or opinionated people. I'm talking about folks who career through life apparently unaware that other people have needs, feelings or thoughts which need consideration. They aren't apparently anxious, because they don't care what you think about their words or actions, however crass they may be. They tend to talk too loudly, don't wait for your reply, invade your space and ignore social conventions. This is the guy on the train (in the quiet carriage) who talks so loudly on his mobile phone that you can't concentrate on what you're reading and it's also him who dives at the last minute into the parking space you've been waiting five minutes for. He is the life and soul of the party and dominates whatever environment is unfortunate enough to include him. He actually does experience anxiety, but only over whether he may not get everything he wants, or whether you may not notice him. I try to avoid these people when I can, but a part of me marvels at what they are able to get away with. Their life strategy seems to work well, at least for them. The lesson they can teach us is clear: we need to care about other people, but *not too much*. If we can be a bit bolder, more adventurous, less vigilant, we're likely to achieve more and enjoy more.

Then there are the 'cool dudes', those people who breeze through situations without an apparent care in the world, facing crises without a hair out of place or breaking into a sweat. Jim never loses his cool, is always in control, has a ready quip to defuse the most awkward situations and, despite not being physically remarkable, seems to attract a wide array of friends of both sexes. How does he do it? While to an extent Jim may be constitutionally confident, with low anxiety levels, mostly his demeanour is achieved by a combination of learning and hard work. He may actually be a lot more anxious than he appears, seeming cool and confident because he needs to gain the approval of others to compensate for feelings of inferiority or inadequacy. I have seen a number of people who appear really cool, calm and confident, but whose insecurity and anxiety is only revealed in the privacy of my consulting room. Don't always believe what you see. On the other hand, even if he was internally lacking confidence in the past, by acting confidently the chances are that Jim will become more confident and less anxious over time, because of the *you become the way that you act* principle (see Chapter 2).

If he really does have low anxiety levels, Jim probably learnt this early on in life. The chances are that his parents were consistently loving and taught him that he was wonderful, whatever he did or didn't achieve. That doesn't mean that he could get away with anything, but that even if he was scolded for laziness or bad behaviour, he was never made to feel bad or inadequate as a person. A difficult balance for parents this: how to teach a kid to strive and to be a good citizen while also learning 'I'm OK'. If Jim's parents weren't able to achieve this balance, he can learn it later on, through kind and loving friendships, relationships and other affirmative experiences. If he is religious, some churches are able to be very supportive and nurturing. Choose carefully though – I have found some of the kindest and some of the meanest people I have ever met in churches.

Most of all, Jim has worked hard at being cool. Most cool dudes put a lot of effort into looking good and acting cool. Calmness and serenity don't drop ready-made from the heavens for most of us; we have to go and find them.

Which brings me to people who are 'Zen'. I don't just mean Buddhist monks and adherents of yoga who are able to lift their foot above their head, although these folks are clearly very good at achieving a state of calmness. I mean all those who are able to meet life on its own terms, to experience it moment by moment, rather than fighting it, railing against it or trying to control every aspect of it. My friend Loretta is able to face trivial reverses, such as playing a bad golf shot, or major hazards, such as a cancer scare, with the same resigned smile and shrug of the shoulders. Has she always been that way? I don't think so. She's worked at it. Can you learn serenity? Yes, you can. Read on …

Part 2
STRATEGIES AND TREATMENTS

5

Managing your anxiety – do this first: lifestyle skills and changes

There is a lot you can do yourself before getting treatment for your anxiety. This doesn't mean you should delay visiting your GP. Many psychological treatments delivered by healthcare providers involve a waiting list and it's just as well to get on it now. But, in the meantime, there's a whole load you can start working on. If you've gone out and bought this book, then it's my guess that either you or someone you care about is suffering from anxiety severe and longstanding enough to cause great suffering and a lack of joy, fulfilment and achievement. That's most of what life is about, so it's certainly worth putting some time and effort into changing what you can. Here are some of the skills and habits that you can teach yourself. They may not seem like much, but they can make a real difference. Do these before or at the same time as you start any specific treatments.

Exercise

There is a wealth of evidence for the anti-anxiety effects of exercise. None of it is a surprise as the physical effects of anxiety are designed to stimulate you to physical activity. Aerobic exercise (anything which puts up your heart rate and gets you a bit out of puff) uses up adrenaline and quietens the hypothalamus (see Chapter 2). In addition, exercise stimulates release of endorphins, leading to greater calmness and wellbeing.

If it's been some time since you've taken regular exercise, you may need to start slowly and possibly get some advice from your doctor, particularly if you have ongoing physical health issues.

But do get started. Presuming you aren't elderly or infirm and you aren't advised otherwise, starting with around half an hour of gentle exercise a day, five times a week, is reasonable. A brisk walk will do it. Increase the time and intensity gradually as you get fitter. You'll need to be quite disciplined about this. There are always good reasons why you haven't got time for exercise, particularly if you have a busy and stressful life, but there has to be a priority given to regular exercise if this is going to work. Before I retired, I used to put on my running gear and go for a short jog every day after work, as my first action after getting home. A prioritized routine is crucial. Don't leave it to a decision on the spot. If you get home after a difficult day at work and ask yourself: 'Shall I put on my kit and go for a jog, or shall I pour myself a gin and tonic and watch my favourite show?', I think I know which decision will prevail and it won't involve pounding the streets.

Exercise is no fun when you're unfit but, if you stick at it, you'll start to find that you enjoy it, as well as noticing a decrease in your anxiety. If you need more structure and purpose, by all means go to the gym, get a trainer, or take up a sport (not just darts or snooker, obviously). Whatever it is, do it regularly.

Habits, routines and balance

This is a generalization but, on the whole, people who suffer with anxiety disorders care a lot. They care about doing the right thing (always) and doing things right (perfectly), about how they are perceived by others and about controlling events so that nothing can go wrong. The trouble is that trying to nail down life and other people is like trying to nail down an armful of eels; you just make a mess and as likely as not hurt yourself.

The result is that little is achieved other than fear and exhaustion. So a crucial starting point in managing anxiety is trying to let go a bit. I know that's not as easy as it sounds but, as I've explained already, if you change the way you operate,

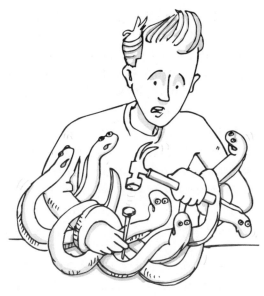

you'll change too. Letting go means doing a bit less, for others as well as yourself. It means checking a bit less often, whatever it is that you check. It means trying a bit less hard at whatever has been your main priority or priorities. It means looking for balance in your life, that is work–life balance but also the balance between your needs and those of others, between rest, exercise and recreation, between doing useful stuff and just blobbing in front of the TV. Everything is about balance. My observation is that many of my anxious patients were so busy trying to do and be everything for everybody that they had no idea how to find a balance in their lives. They care so much for and about everyone else that they neglect themselves, their own needs and wishes. So that's where you need to start. It's not that you're more important than anyone else, but you do matter just as much.

The best way to get balance in your life is to develop a routine. In constructing this, you need to put in the stuff you really value first. I'll illustrate using a parable. A teacher shows his students a large bell jar. He then puts rocks into it, so that they reach the top of the jar. 'Is the jar full?' he asks. 'Yes,' replies a student. The professor then pours some pebbles around the rocks, again up to the top of the jar. 'Is the jar full now?' he asks. 'Yes,' answers another student. The teacher then pours sand around the rocks and pebbles. 'Each time you thought the jar was full, there was in fact space for more,' he points out. 'The bell jar is your life. The sand is the stuff that has to get done, the chores and necessities, bills, washing and the like. The pebbles are the things and people you care about, your job, looking after family and friends, health and so forth. The rocks are the stuff that makes your life have real meaning, what it's really for: hobbies, interests, loves and passions. I put the rocks in first and everything fitted around them.' He then takes another bell jar and fills it with sand. There is no space left to fit in any pebbles or rocks. 'That's what happens if you don't find balance in your life and don't put what gives your life meaning first,' concludes the Prof. He's right. An optional postscript to this story has the teacher opening a can of beer and pouring it into the first bell jar. It pours over the rocks, pebbles and sand, just filling to the top of the jar. 'This demonstrates,' declares the sage, 'that however full your life may be, there's always room for a beer.' Just one though.

So develop a routine with the good, fun, enriching stuff put in first. Make sure that it's balanced, with a bit of everything rather than seeking perfection in any one area. Life isn't perfect and you shouldn't try to make it so. For me, very good is better than perfect, because it's real and sustainable.

Pace yourself. Life is a marathon, not a sprint. The competitor who runs the first mile of the marathon in four minutes isn't going to win the race.

Try to free yourself from the need to please others or to gain their approval all the time. Obviously, we all need to take account of the feelings, opinions and advice of those around us, but the day you first manage to let someone be unhappy with you without trying to make it right is the day you'll be free and start to get control of your anxiety.

Make sure that your habits are those that you'd be happy to recommend to your dearest friend. If not, if they are such that it would be unreasonable or unkind to expect them of anyone else, you're engaging in double standards. Think again and change your habits.

Caffeine and alcohol

Caffeine is a stimulant of the same type (though less potent) as amphetamines ('speed'). It hangs around in your system for several hours after drinking a cup of coffee or tea and, if you drink several cups in a day, you'll be getting a build-up of caffeine in your system. More so if you drink Red Bull, and most colas and energy drinks also contain caffeine. Many anxious people drink a lot of coffee and tea to get them going, not realizing that it could be making their anxiety worse.

Then they have a few drinks in the evening to switch off. The trouble is that alcohol reverses its own effect with regular heavy use. The drinks you had last night will be making you more anxious today, even if you didn't have enough to give you a hangover. As little as a pint of ordinary strength beer has been shown to increase anxiety the next day by enough to be measurable, but it's if you're drinking two or more times that level regularly that the increase in your anxiety really becomes significant. There will be a slow ratcheting up of your anxiety over time. You may well not be aware this is happening, because each time you have a drink you feel better (for a short time). Don't be fooled, regular heavy drinking makes you anxious. Refer back to Figure 2 in Chapter 2 for an illustration of this process.

If you have been consuming a lot of caffeine or alcohol or both for a long time, don't stop suddenly, as you'll feel worse for a week or two if you do and stopping daily heavy drinking suddenly without medical support is potentially dangerous. But do cut down, slowly but steadily, looking to get off these drugs over a few weeks. I would then recommend avoiding caffeine and limiting yourself to one drink at weekends only, at least until you have your anxiety well under control.

Relaxation

Relaxation exercises can be immensely powerful if persevered with, allowing you to bring your level of arousal down a great deal. There is a long way to go if you're severely anxious, so it'll take time, but in the end it'll be worth it. This exercise is the same one that appears in my earlier books, so you may be familiar with it already. There are many variations on this theme and the thing is to find the one that works best for you. There are several relaxation exercises commercially available as audio files, on CD, flash drive or other spoken word media. Others get benefit from yoga techniques learnt in a group setting. Some find that following a written set of instructions helps them better, by allowing them to do the exercise at their own pace with their own mental imagery. What follows is just one example of such a technique, but one that many of my most anxious patients have found helpful.

Whichever way you choose, the essential point is that it needs a lot of practice. Though a few people pick it up very quickly, for the majority relaxation exercises are a total waste of time *to begin with*. They don't work straight away, leading many to become disillusioned and give up on them. Some people even feel worse at the beginning, because doing anything and having it fail tends to make you feel tense.

Persevere, because when you really master the technique you will find that it changes your life. You're doing it not to get benefit from it yet, but as an investment in your future. The people who get benefit from relaxation exercises are those who put them top of their list of priorities and practise for at least half an hour every day, come hell or high water. If you hear that a meteor is going to vaporize your town in 24 hours, by all means take flight for the hills, but not until you've done your relaxation practice.

Looking back, I did relaxation exercises every day for over two years, not because I was unusually anxious most of the time but because I suffered a panic attack in a crucial exam at medical school, which threatened to halt my career before it had started. I learnt then, because I had to, that there is no limit to how good you can get at relaxation, but that it takes a lot of consistent practice. I'll tell you the full story of this episode in Chapter 9, in the Panic Disorder section. Here's the exercise I learnt and which changed my life.

A relaxation exercise

Spend 20–30 minutes on this exercise.

1 Find a suitable place to relax. A bed or easy chair is ideal, but anywhere will do, preferably quiet and private. Once you are good enough at the exercise to find it useful, do it when you go to bed.
2 Try to clear your mind of thoughts as far as you can.
3 Take three very slow, very deep breaths (10 to 15 seconds to breathe in and out once).
4 Imagine a neutral object. An example may be the number 1. Don't choose any object or figure with emotional significance, such as a ring or a person. Let it fill your mind. See it in your mind's eye, give it a colour, try to see it in 3-D and repeat it to yourself under your breath, many times over. Continue until it fills your mind.
5 Slowly change to imagine yourself in a quiet, peaceful and pleasant place or situation. This may be a favourite place or situation, or a pleasant scene from your past. Be there and notice all the feelings, in each sense. See it, feel it, hear it, smell it and taste it. Spend some time there.
6 Slowly change to be aware of your body. Notice any tension in your body. Take each group of muscles in turn and tense, then relax them two or three times each. Include fingers, hands, arms, shoulders, neck, face, chest, tummy, buttocks,

thighs, legs, feet and toes. Be aware of the feeling of relaxation in contrast to how the tense muscles felt. When complete, spend some time in this relaxed state. If you aren't relaxed, don't worry; you're just practising for now.

7 Slowly get up and go about your business if you're doing the exercise during the day. If it's bedtime, just lie in bed until you drop off to sleep (this is when you're good at it, to begin with remember it may not work).

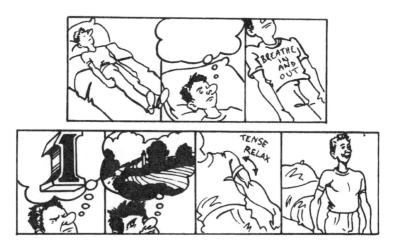

At step 5, I want to emphasize that this isn't simply visualization. It is a *multi-sensory experience*. Let me demonstrate. You are imagining yourself on a beautiful Caribbean beach. Lovely. But that isn't enough. Which direction is the wind coming from? Is it constant or puffy? What does it feel like when the sun goes behind a cloud? Does it get cooler? What does hot sun on sand smell of and what is the smell of your suntan lotion? Is the sand soft or hard? How do the waves sound? What does your drink taste of? How far back does the grass start? Are the palm trees small, stumpy palms or tall coconut palms? If they are coconut palms, are the coconuts brown or green?

You need to be there in every sense. This takes quite a lot of practice.

Don't hurry this procedure and remember to practise. It will work and, when it does, you'll have much more control over your anxiety.

Sleep

This can be a tricky area, because many anxiety sufferers have difficulty getting to sleep, but there are things you can do. If sleep is a major problem for you, please read my book *Beating Insomnia Without Really Trying* (Sheldon Press), which has much more detailed advice than I can include here. For now, I just want to emphasize that improving your sleep is an important step in dealing with anxiety and to touch on three principles that are central to sleeping well.

First, develop a constant routine. Try to have meals, other routines and bedtime at roughly the same time each day. Sleep is governed by circadian rhythms and you develop these by keeping the timing of your daily routines as constant as possible.

Second, let there be darkness. Turn the lights down later in the evening and, when it comes to bedtime, do not have any LCD displays operating in the bedroom. That means leaving your mobile phone and tablet in the sitting room. No TV in the bedroom. Put a 40-watt bulb (or less) in your bedside lamp. Don't use a backlit e-reader. Your brain interprets the blue light from these devices as daylight and a signal to wake up.

Last, don't take work or other tasks to bed with you. You can't be alert and sleepy at the same time, so the alertness needed for a work task will stop you getting to sleep for some time after you've completed it. Try only to think of nice things that make you feel calm at bedtime. If worries, hassles or tasks keep popping into your head after you've switched the light out, keep a notepad and pencil beside your bed and jot down the thoughts as they arrive. Have a pre-set time in the morning when you look at the notepad and consider what you've written. At night your brain will then believe that it doesn't need to resolve the issues immediately and will allow you to forget them for now. You've physically moved the issues from your brain onto paper and, from there, to a time period the next day.

Problem solving

Again, you will recognize this section from my other books, because problem solving is a crucial skill for those trying to overcome stress-related conditions of all kinds. Learn how to organize problems and you're more than halfway to resolving them. If your anxiety comes from you feeling overwhelmed by a sea of conflicting and apparently insoluble issues, you need to get organized, starting now.

The trouble with problems is that they don't come one at a time or when you're ready to receive them, but at the most inopportune moments and, like London buses, several at once. Many of them conflict with each other so, if you solve one, you feel you'll make another worse. The whole thing seems like a gigantic mess and you feel out of control, so you try to deal with everything at once, resulting in your brain becoming scrambled and nothing being achieved. You get irritable with your spouse, resulting in him becoming grumpy, disengaged and unsupportive. Now he is part of the problem too.

The principle of problem solving is simple: take a set of problems or one big problem and split it up into smaller, bite-size pieces. Let's take an example. You're in a financial mess. The problem is too big to manage, so split it up:

1 I'm above my overdraft limit at the bank.
2 My creditors are beginning to issue threats.
3 My outgoings are more than my income.
4 I have a lot of debtors who show no sign of paying what they owe me.
5 The interest rate is rising, meaning my mortgage payments are increasing.

6 My car is old and getting more expensive to run.

7 Christmas is a month away and I can't afford presents for the kids.

Now you have a better-defined set of problems to consider. Take each one separately, in turn, and brainstorm some actions which you could take. Include all the ideas you come up with: the good, the less good and the apparently ridiculous. It's remarkable how often ideas that seem wacky turn out to be strokes of genius. So, for problem 1 above a possible list might be:

a) Arrange a meeting with my bank manager to request an increase in my overdraft limit.

b) Explain that the problem is of cash flow and that I'm in the process of resolving it.

c) Take out a short-term loan.

d) Borrow from friends/relatives.

e) Cut out items of expenditure (refer to separate expenditure list).

f) Ignore it and hope it'll all go away.

g) Try to get more overtime at work.

h) Sell the house and downsize.

i) Look for a job with a better salary.

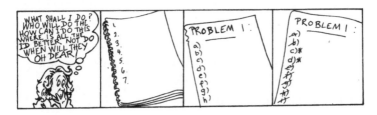

Now think through each option in turn and rule out those which won't work. Maybe talk them through with someone you trust.

Go through this process for each of problems 1–7. You'll then come up with a list of action points, some of which will come up more than once. Gather this list together and number them in order of priority. Act on them one at a time, ticking each one off as you action it. Be realistic in what you set yourself. Don't try to do everything in a day. It's important that you act in a way that is sustainable and doesn't lead to exhaustion. Slow and steady is the way. If you pace yourself, the process of working through action points is satisfying and empowering. Now you're doing everything you can to resolve your problems.

Of course, following this structure doesn't make them disappear overnight, but it does give you some control and reduces the fear that was escalating while you were avoiding them.

Time management, prioritizing and the 3× multiplier

I used to rush around a lot, overfilling my day and not always achieving a lot. Now that I've retired, I can't say that my life is too busy (don't tell my publishers that as then they'll expect me to deliver book manuscripts on time). My wife is still working and I see her struggle to fit everything in. I've developed a rule of thumb, which applies well to her and also, I think, to most busy people, which I call the 3x multiplier. If Laura says 'I'll be finished in 20 minutes,' it'll be an hour; if she says an hour, it'll be 3 hours, and so on. Tasks take longer than you think. So, if you think you have just enough time to juggle all the tasks you've set yourself this week, you probably haven't. You'll need to prioritize. And remember that you have to plan in some downtime and 'you' time as well.

For many anxiety sufferers, the main problem is becoming overwhelmed by the sea of problems and priorities which they face. You rush around in ever decreasing circles trying to do everything at once and getting nowhere. So stop, make yourself a cup of decaf tea and take the 30 minutes which you don't have to make a time plan. The one illustrated below is a weekly time plan for a single business executive without children. Yours will probably look very different, but the principle is very important. Organizing your time so that you're doing things

	Monday	Tuesday	Wednesday	Thursday	Friday	Saturday	Sunday
9 am				filing	deliver report	shopping	↑
10 am	admin meeting	spare for crisis and problems	personal work	computer work	travel		
11 am					meet with client		
12 am				prepare report			
1 pm		L	U N	C H			rest
2 pm	personal work	travel	presentation	meeting about report	travel	rest	↓
3 pm		meeting	rest		personal work		
4 pm			travel	admin	prepare next week's time plan		
5 pm							
Evening	rest	prepare presentation	late meeting	going out	rest	theatre	

Figure 4 A time plan

together which can be done in one place and building in breaks and spaces for unforeseen contingencies will make your life run a lot more smoothly and reduce your stress levels significantly.

Before all the mothers with small children throw this book against the wall, let me say, I know – being a parent, particularly if you have little in the way of support, is well-nigh impossible. No time plan will change that. But do remember that being a 'good enough' parent is better for your kids than trying to be perfect. Sitting them in front of the TV for half an hour while you put your feet up isn't going to do them any harm. Your children matter a lot, but so do you.

Avoiding avoidance

I will expand on this later when I talk about dealing with phobias, but there's a general principle for all anxiety here which you need to start working on straight away. It's natural that you should want to avoid what makes you anxious, or to avoid everything if you're anxious all the time. But that makes it worse. Avoidance is what keeps anxiety going. I don't mean that you have to plunge headlong into the situations which terrify you the most all at once, but you do need to start doing a little bit. Baby steps. For example, a young man, John, is anxious about talking with women, though he would dearly love to have a girlfriend. I'm not saying that John should immediately force himself to go to parties, especially where he doesn't know many people and especially not in a situation where he has accepted a lift to and from the party from someone else, so that he's trapped at the event until his driver chooses to leave. But if some folks from work including a couple of women are going out for a drink after work and John is invited, he should go. He should explain that he only has half an hour as he's expecting an important call at home. If, at the pub, he only manages to say a couple of words, that isn't a failure. It's a triumph. He's started to face his fear and he can continue a little at a time, so long as he doesn't give in to his tendency to judge himself negatively or go back to avoiding his fears.

Remember, what you've been avoiding for years is going to be your area of least competence. That's inevitable. You'll only get better at it through practice and sympathetic acceptance of your own limitations (for now). Think about how a good teacher encourages a child to learn. She doesn't shout at the kid when he makes a mistake. She points out what he did wrong, then encourages him to try again. When I was a child, my Maths master used to hit us with a stick when we got a sum wrong. As a result, not one of my class of very bright kids went on to study Mathematics or Physics at University. Punishment only ensures avoidance, and harsh self-criticism is punishment. So treat yourself kindly as you edge very gradually towards your fears.

Thought stopping

Negative thoughts become habitual and ingrained. Often, they get in the way of rational thoughts and prevent you from

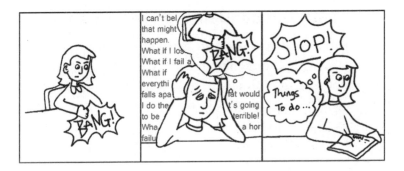

making good decisions. You may be aware of this and try to chase these unhelpful thoughts away, but they keep popping back into your head, like an unwanted pop-up message on your computer. That's when you need a method of stopping these thoughts in their tracks. This one can work well with practice.

When you're on your own in a place where sound doesn't travel too far, make a sudden loud noise, such as banging the table or dropping something loud on a hard surface. Remember the jolt that this sudden sound gives you. When you find yourself mulling over an unwanted repetitive thought, bring this memory into your mind, allowing it to give you a jolt. Say sharply to yourself: *'Stop'*. This does not have to be out loud, but imagine yourself saying it sharply and loudly. This interruption will give you a gap in your repetitive thoughts. Take advantage of this gap by substituting a more helpful and appropriate thought. Or start a relaxation exercise or go and do something which requires active concentration. You may need to repeat this procedure more than once and, like anything, it may take some practice to work well in the most difficult situations, which is when it's needed. I know that some people use a rubber band around their wrist which they ping in order to stop repetitive thoughts. If that works for you, fine, but I have some misgivings about inflicting pain on yourself, whatever the purpose.

Sharing and dependence on reassurance

A problem shared is a problem halved. Everyone knows that. While this saying is certainly true, it needs to be employed with judgement. Like most things, reassurance can be addictive if used habitually as your only way of dealing with anxiety. Sometimes you need to spend time with your anxiety rather than compulsively seeking someone out to chase it away for you.

Say you fear that your kids may pick up some dreadful bug which the press says has been brought into the country, with three people hospitalized and one child at your daughter's school being suspected of having contracted it. You can talk to your spouse about it, and a friend who has some medical knowledge. You may even seek reassurance from your GP. All OK so far. But what if you're not reassured? How many friends should you share your fears with? Only a few at most and only wise ones who aren't prone to exaggeration. Unfortunately, some folks love to peddle worrying rumours. And remember the rule: the degree of a person's certainty is usually in inverse proportion to their wisdom and knowledge. How often should you seek your spouse's reassurance? When anything changes or any new news item emerges. Otherwise once every few days maximum, with the aim of gradually reducing the frequency with which you seek the comfort of his reassurance.

Do share your worries, but keep an eye on your dependence on reassurance. You need to internalize some of the reassuring words you have heard and to start repeating them to yourself. If you feel that you can't do this, that you are totally dependent on outside reassurance and that this reliance is taking over your life, you may need to go and talk to your GP if you haven't done so already. This is where professional help (see later) comes in. Hopefully you're already on a waiting list for therapy but, if you aren't, now is the time to get started.

6

Managing your anxiety – second phase: changing your outlook

Anxiety is horrible. It's not surprising that you are anxious about feeling anxious, as fear is one of the worst kinds of suffering and it's even less surprising that you should try to avoid it. Unfortunately, as I suggested in the last chapter, avoiding what makes you anxious and trying to avoid the feeling itself only makes it worse. You can't do battle with anxiety or escape from it; it's like trying to fight with fog or running from it.

But you can take charge. Your life and the decisions you make belong to you, not your anxiety. You can decide on a strategy for managing your life which takes account of your fear, but is not ruled by it. What would you do in the situation you face were it not for your fear? What would your fearless friend do in your place? These are good indicators of the way forward. While fear is frightening, it can't actually do you any harm in the short term. What you do to avoid it can.

So don't try too hard to avoid your fear, but don't fight it either. *Accept it*, then go about your business *as you choose to*. Decide on your strategies, using the advice of wise friends and, if you have one, your therapist, as well as things you learn from this book, and your own sense of what a less fearful you would do. Obviously, there is a limit to how useful fearlessness can be, as I explained in Chapter 4. We're not talking about a lack of fear here, but a degree of fear in balance with the situation you're in.

So you thought I was going to tell you how to fight your fear? I'm not. I'm advising you to accept your fear, staying with it rather than avoiding it and, in time, learning how to manage it. Over time, probably with the help of medication, therapy and the strategies in this book, your anxiety, like fog, will lift, but you won't be able to say in retrospect when it happened, it'll just be that the fog is now only a gentle mist. From time to time the fog may descend again, but each time less dense and for a shorter time.

In this chapter, I've listed some of the changes in how you see things and do things that are going to be needed for you to get back in charge of your life.

Social skills

Life is a lot easier for those who are lucky enough to be socially confident and skilled. If you've suffered from anxiety for a long time, especially if some of your fear centres around social situations, you're unlikely to be one of that group. Skill comes from practice and you won't have had a lot of that. So your starting point needs to be accepting where you're starting from. The fact that you're not the life and soul of the party and that you don't have a host of devoted friends *isn't your fault*. It's an inevitable result of your anxiety.

But that doesn't mean that you have to accept how you are. It's time to make a start. As I've already explained, it's best to start slowly, with something not too demanding. If you've been almost completely isolated, spending nearly all your time in your room, then meeting with someone you know in a Starbucks for 20 minutes, or even just saying 'hi' to the postman is enough. It's a start.

Watch people who are good at social interaction. It's not that you're going to be able to emulate them any time soon, but you can pick up some tips. How do they start the conversation with someone they've never met? What sort of things do they talk about? Do you notice how they ask more questions of the person they're talking to, rather than talking about themselves? And how they look for common ground, like sports they follow or TV programmes they've watched?

Then have a go, in as undemanding a setting as you can come up with.

Then comes the most important part. *Fail.* I mean that you won't be very good at it. The interaction will seem awkward and gauche to you. Of course it will; you're out of practice. *Forgive yourself* for this and reframe the experience. It's a triumph. For the first time in ages you've faced your fear and your weakest area. That's admirable. The fact it didn't go well is irrelevant. You did it. Don't allow any self-talk along the lines of 'I'm so stupid, I should have said …'. That's bullying and unhelpful. You wouldn't say it to anyone else, so don't say it to yourself.

Now learn from the experience. What could you have done differently? What went well? Next time, are you going to seek out a similar situation, something easier or more demanding? Take it slowly.

Then try again. Not straight away. Maybe tomorrow. You don't need your life to be a constant series of trials, but you do need to get some social practice. Plan out what you're going to try next. As always, seek support and advice if you need to.

Developing social skills is all about practice, treating yourself well when you fail and not giving up.

If you want to read more about how to improve social skills, try *Conversation Skills for the Shy: How to easily talk to anyone* by Emma Watkins or *Coping with Shyness and Social Anxiety* by Ruth Searle.

Managing family and friends

Because you're anxious you lack confidence and that, in turn, makes it easy to take advantage of you. Family and friends tend to be the worst offenders. It's not that they are mean or intend to be unkind, but it's just human nature. We tend to ask more of those who have difficulty saying 'no' than we do of those who are more confident and assertive. So anxious people sometimes become overloaded by trying to please those around them.

The opposite can also be true. Loved ones hate to see you suffer, so they often stop including you in things, lest doing so might make you uncomfortable. Unwittingly, they can end up making you increasingly isolated and lacking in confidence.

In the end, constructing an effective boundary which has you included but not put-upon is going to be down to you. This is going to mean you trying less hard to please others and trying harder to work out and express your own needs. When you've worked out what you really want (not what's easiest, but the point you want to reach), you'll need to talk to those who care about you, explaining what you need from them. If you don't know what that is, talk to the person who you trust most. How can family and friends best help you? This is quite a turn-around, as I suspect you've not spent a lot of time up until now thinking about what your needs are. Most of your time has been spent either avoiding your fears or the disapproval of those around you.

Understand and accept your anxiety

As I explained in Part 1, anxiety produces a range of physical symptoms. These are natural, your body adapting to perceived threat. These symptoms are part of the 'fight-or-flight' reaction. *So don't fight them.* Battling your symptoms only fuels them. Your physical symptoms aren't going to harm you in the short term and the best way to overcome them in the long term is to *accept them.* However unpleasant and scary your symptoms may be, *let them be.* Understand what they are: a normal physical reaction. That doesn't mean you can't do whatever you are able to in order to deal with your anxiety; that's what this book is about. Just don't rail against its effects. By all means go to your doctor to get a physical check-up, but when you are told that your symptoms are caused by anxiety, try to accept this advice. Understanding and acceptance really are the most important principles in dealing with anxiety.

Let them be

This principle of acceptance extends beyond your symptoms. What about your thoughts? You may be painfully aware that some of them would seem crazy if people could see inside your head. Let me reassure you though: your crazy thoughts aren't crazy. Everyone has them. Believe me, if you could see inside my head, particularly when the current leader of the free world is on the TV, you'd have me locked up. But this doesn't mean I'm dangerous – I wouldn't hurt anyone. Thoughts are just thoughts, unless they are accompanied by intent. Indeed, some anxious people find the most shocking thing they can think of playing repeatedly in their head. So if, for example, for you child abuse is the most shocking thing you can think of, that is what will be the subject of your ruminations. That doesn't mean that you are at risk of abusing children, far from it. That's the last thing you'd do. Crazy, abhorrent thoughts, in the absence of any problems other than anxiety, are just symptoms and have no meaning. So let them play. Ignore them as you would a naughty attention-seeking kid who wants to shock you. Don't be shocked, just get on with whatever you're doing and treat the upsetting thoughts as the irrelevance they are.

Then there are the ordinary negative thoughts and worries that dominate the lives of folks who suffer from anxiety. What to do with them? The answer is let them fly by like a flock of birds. Watch them as they go past, but don't engage with them. Let them pass through your mind on their way to somewhere else. They don't belong to you, so don't hold on to them. I'll come back to this in the next chapter when I discuss mindfulness.

People can be a real problem. For me, it's bombastic bullies I can't endure. I find myself wanting to prick the bubble of their nastiness and arrogance. But then I realize that the problem is me, not them. Bullies have always existed and always will. Why should it be my role to change them? Most of these folks like

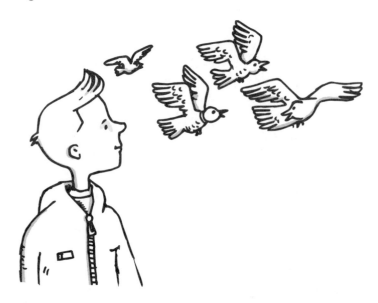

nothing better than a scrap, verbal or physical. Better to leave them be and find someone less tiresome to focus on. The same is true for anyone you find toxic. Try not to engage with them unless you have to. If you're put in a position where you have to fight your corner, as sometimes you have to with bullies and other toxic types, do so as well as you can, but be realistic. Toxic people are better at being toxic than you are at resisting them, as they've been practising their whole lives. In general, when you can, accept people as you find them, the nasty as well as the nice. But avoid the nasty ones when you can. This is about the only type of avoidance that I recommend in dealing with anxiety.

So accept your symptoms, your thoughts and people. But also try to accept life as you find it, rather than as it ought to be. Life isn't fair and never will be but, from time to time, it gives you a gift you haven't earned. At other times it deals you an undeserved blow. Every happy person I've ever met has succeeded in accepting the ups and downs of their life. They experience their lives rather than trying to dictate how they should be and demanding of life that it be fair. You'll know by now that I'm a golfer. I've seen many playing partners who get a bad break and focus on the injustice of it for the rest of the round, resulting in their game going to pieces. In their grumbling discontent, they ignore the fact that on the first hole their ball, which was headed out of bounds, hit a tree and bounced back into the fairway. Apparently only the bad breaks count. Other golfers just shrug their shoulders and get on with the next shot, whether their break was good or bad. They usually win. Who said that golf was supposed to be fair? In that, it's an excellent metaphor for life.

This type of serene acceptance of life on its own terms is hard. As with everything else, be honest with yourself and keep trying. There is no secret to serenity (other than God, if you believe in Him), there's just trying over and over again. I think it was David Bailey who said that the secret of taking a great photograph is to take a lot of photographs. The same holds true for attempts to gain acceptance and serenity.

There is one change that you can make straight away though. That is to make fewer value judgements. That is of things, people or yourself being 'good', 'bad', 'clever', 'ignorant', 'admirable', 'pathetic', 'weak', 'strong', 'fine person', 'jerk' or whatever. These judgements tell us less about the world than about the person making the judgement. They do harm to the judged, particularly if you are both the judge and the judged. So try to judge less, others but particularly yourself.

Recognize false alarms

As I've already explained, it's not just that anxiety causes symptoms. Symptoms also generate anxiety, leading to the setting up of a vicious cycle. So it's important for you to recognize these 'false alarms'. Note down the physical anxiety symptoms that have made you scared before. A racing heart beat doesn't mean you're having a heart attack. Breathlessness doesn't mean you're going to suffocate. Stomach pains, nausea, retching, bloating or other abdominal symptoms don't mean you have life-threatening pathology in your gut. Numbness or tingling in your fingers or toes, dizziness or light-headedness don't mean you're having a stroke. If you suffer with anxiety, the chances are that these symptoms are related to your anxiety rather than anything else. You have probably suffered these symptoms before. If you have, what was the outcome? If it wasn't a heart attack last time, it probably isn't this time either and, if the symptoms eventually settled of their own accord before, they will again. By all means write out this paragraph and read it the next time you get anxious about a 'false alarm'. Of course, some judgement is required here. You can't ignore all symptoms, but if the one in question has already been explained by your GP as not indicating physical disease and nothing else has changed, accept the reassurance you have already received.

You may be aware that the symptoms you feel building are of a panic attack, but not be reassured by this because panic attacks are so unpleasant. You're panicky about panicking. But *it will pass and it will do you no harm.* The solution to your symptoms (I know, I do go on a bit) is to accept them.

Reduce checking activities

People suffering with obsessive-compulsive disorder (not dealt with in this book) tend to have the greatest difficulty in limiting the time they spend in trying to reassure themselves through checking. Next come those with specific phobias. But, in fact, most people with anxiety states of any kind tend to spend an excessive amount of time in checking on their fears. The trouble is that it doesn't work. The more you check, the more you need to check, because you're checking to reassure yourself that what you fear isn't happening and, as I explained earlier, reassurance is addictive. So you need to set strict limits to how much time you spend on checking activities.

In Chapter 5, I gave the example of you being anxious about a bug at your daughter's school which has led to one child being admitted to hospital. Is it OK to ring the school to find out more details and get advice? Yes. Is it OK to phone your GP for advice? Yes. Is it OK to do some research on the infection on the internet? Possibly, though I have misgivings about internet-based research. Beware the abundance of nonsense on the web – stick to reputable medical websites – and put a limit on how long you spend trawling the internet. Is it OK to keep an eye on your daughter to look out for the relevant symptoms? Yes. But what about phoning the school for updates twice a day, taking your daughter to the GP for checkups every day, hovering constantly over her and taking her temperature hourly, keeping her indoors 24/7 or spending eight hours a day trawling the internet for horror stories about school infections? No, that helps nobody and only increases your anxiety. You need to talk to your spouse or partner, or family and friends, decide on an appropriate limit to your checking and then stick to it. This will be very hard at first, but easier as time goes on.

Rescript and reframe

It's often not the thing itself which we are most scared of, but how we react to it. Say you have to do a presentation at work. You fear public speaking and have avoided it whenever possible. As a result, you have little practice or confidence at it. You could avoid it by finding some reason to pull out or by going off sick. But you go ahead and do the presentation. It isn't fluent, it is no masterpiece, you stutter a bit, leave one part out and you are painfully aware that you are flushed and sweating, but you complete it. Many of my patients respond to an event like this by being harshly self-critical, when what is needed is praise. Praise which is well earned. It's easy if it's easy, but this was difficult and you did it. The colleague who breezes up to the podium and gives a polished masterclass doesn't deserve the praise, because she's just done what is easy for her. You do, because you did what is hard for you.

There are at least three scripts here that you need to change. First, the future script: I'm about to do the presentation. It has to be perfect. Everyone will judge me. I'll break down and it will be a humiliating disaster. Change this to something like: I'm not confident at this, so I won't be perfect or a star, but I can just go through the motions and get it done. That will be a success, however well or badly I present. I'll be anxious, so I will probably sweat and flush, but I won't be the first who has shown nerves, so it really doesn't matter.

Another way of looking at future scripts is *reframing*. A psychologist colleague likes to ask his clients to draw three scenarios for how the situation they face will play out: the worst, the best and the most likely. In our example, the worst scenario might be you coming to a grinding halt, fainting or vomiting and being carried off the podium while everyone laughs at you. Likelihood: about the same as of me being selected to play rugby for England. The best: carrying off a perfect and memorable tour-de-force. Fractionally more likely, but not much. The most likely: you'll get through, not perfectly, but ok. Folks may realize you're nervous and that this isn't really your thing, but so what? Chances: very likely. Accept the likely outcome, it's probably what will happen. This sort of reframing is very powerful if you get in the habit of doing it.

Second, the past script: That was a disaster. I was awful, a blushing sweaty mess. I should have done so much better. No, you shouldn't, that's neither fair nor realistic. Getting through it was the best you could do. You succeeded.

Third, the audience script: They must have all been thinking what an idiot I am. They'll all be laughing at me, because I was in such a state. I bet Ian will start calling me 'sweaty man'. Now, I can't promise that Ian won't come up with something cruel like that, as there are a few people who get off on taunting people.

If he does, tell him to go to blazes as profanely as you like, then avoid him wherever possible. But don't buy into his taunt; it isn't true. You did well and you only sweated because you were understandably anxious. And the vast majority of your decent colleagues, while realizing that you were anxious, won't judge you for it. Apart from anything else, they'll be more concerned with their own issues than with making harsh judgements about you.

There are hundreds of examples around this theme. The point is that you need to recognize the repeated scripts in your life from which you read. It is really important that you change them. You can start doing that now, talking to wise friends and family about your habitual scripts if you need to, even before you start in any formal therapy.

More on this in the section on cognitive-behavioural therapy (CBT) in Chapter 7, which is all about changing your unhelpful thought patterns.

Deal with shame

This follows on from rescripting and I've already talked about how you need to challenge your tendency to excessive self-criticism, but I believe I need to emphasize it further. There has been a lot of research showing how destructive the emotion of shame can be. While it is natural that we should be ashamed if we've done something wrong, you haven't done anything wrong by being anxious. You are who you are and you've reached this point in your life not through badness or malice, but by having the experiences which you've had, particularly at formative times in your life. Do you think that someone who has a deformed limb should be ashamed? I don't. So why should you be ashamed that you have an overactive amygdala (see Chapter 1).

This is important, because shame leads to avoidance. The alcoholic ashamed of his drinking escapes his shame by denying his problem and getting drunk. The only way he is going to achieve recovery from his addiction is to recognize that he has a disease and that if he accepts treatment, he will deserve to be proud, not ashamed. Exactly the same is true for someone suffering from anxiety. Shame can make you deny your problems and avoid them. Don't be ashamed, you don't deserve it, but do take action to deal with the problem. You've started by reading this book. Start by being proud of yourself for that.

Prepare, but try less and care less

In so many ways, my anxious patients were a pleasure to work with. Apart from anything else, they *tried so hard*. At everything. This included following my suggestions to the letter, taking their medication regularly and on time, going to every therapy session, carrying out homework assignments and anything else they were asked to do. If anything, they tried a bit too hard. This can be a major problem, because twisting every nerve and sinew isn't compatible with bringing down your level of arousal, which is what we're after. So your task is to prepare well, to learn and practise the skills and strategies outlined in this book and by your therapist, but then to act as if you *don't try too hard*.

The professional golfer Freddie Couples mastered this strategy. He had to, as he suffered from the affliction all golfers dread: the 'yips'. This twitch as you're trying to putt results from tension in the hands caused by the pressure of trying to hole a putt. The closer you are to the hole, the worse the yips become, as 'nobody misses a two-footer'. Well, yes they do actually, and fear that you will do so brings on the tension that causes the yips. You can still watch Freddie on the Seniors Tour. You'll see him strolling nonchalantly around the green, seemingly without a care in the world, but clearly taking in all the information he can about slope, pace, grain, wind and anything else that could affect how the ball will roll. Then, when his turn comes, he just steps up and hits the putt. Whether he holes it or misses, his reaction is the same. He just keeps going as if he's out for a Sunday afternoon stroll, cool and unperturbed. He has persuaded himself that *he doesn't care* whether the ball goes in the hole or not, just that he makes a good stroke. This released the stress he had experienced with putting and made him a much better player. I think Freddie can teach us a lot about how to manage stress and anxiety. By all means prepare as well as you can, but then try to *try less hard* and try to *care less*. Just go through the motions.

Paradoxical injunction, massed practice and making it worse

Extensions to the principle of trying less hard are paradoxical injunction and massed practice. A therapist using paradoxical injunction tells his client to do the opposite of what is desired. This is done when the sufferer is so dominated by resistance that more conventional therapeutic efforts are thwarted. A patient of mine had a compulsion to check door knobs to ensure the doors were properly closed (details slightly changed to preserve anonymity). He did so every minute from dawn to dusk, to such an extent that he wore a hole in his right hand, which was getting infected. Nothing could stop his checking, as he felt compelled to resist anything diverting him from his task. So we told him to check *more often*. Every thirty seconds, or even more. He no longer bust a gut trying to resist his urge to check the door handles. As a result, his anxiety reduced and, with it, the frequency of his checking.

This 'paradoxical' principle is used with caution in practice. It doesn't always work, but it can do so if the stress of resisting your anxious impulses is feeding your anxiety. Don't keep going too long if it isn't working and, if in doubt, wait until you can get professional advice.

Expanding on this idea, it can be useful to engage in 'massed practice'. Say you are anxious that you might have picked up an infection that the press reports is in your area and is dangerous.

You find yourself checking your temperature every half an hour. You realize that this is only feeding your anxiety, so you try very hard to resist reaching for the thermometer. This is only making you more stressed and a vicious cycle of increasing fear is set up. Maybe try taking your temperature continuously, every few seconds. Carry on until either you're exhausted or feeling that the activity is ridiculous and are inclined to stop. This may reduce the urge to check your temperature, at least for a while.

Or, try to make the symptom which is tormenting you worse. Say you are trying desperately to calm down so that your irritable bowel will settle. You're trying so hard to be calm that you are getting increasingly wound up and your IBS is worse than ever. So stop trying to make it better. *Try to make it worse.* Try to ramp up your anxiety so that your IBS will be the worst it has ever been. The chances are that stopping efforts to overcome your symptoms will lead to a reduction in your anxiety and thus an improvement in your bowels.

Isn't it strange how life so often works like that? It gives you what you're after just when you stop trying for it. I've had many people consult me who are desperate to find a loving life partner, only to suffer one failed or abusive relationship after another, or no relationship at all. I always worked on the same thing with them, which was to enable them to feel better about themselves and comfortable with being alone. Time after time with these folks, as they were starting to feel really good about themselves and being single, their life partner would show up, just at the point when he or she wasn't needed. That may be life being perverse, but more likely it is that being really comfortable in yourself is very attractive to good, loving people and puts off those who would like to take advantage of you.

I think the same is often true of anxiety. It goes away when you stop trying to make it go away.

These strategies may or may not work for you, but it's worth being aware of them in any case. Don't keep going with them for a long time if they seem to be making things worse. It can be difficult to decide how long is long enough. Talk to someone wise who you trust if you need to. Then wait until you can talk to a mental health professional before deciding what to do next.

Look for opportunity not fairness

Every happy person I've ever met is good at this. Most anxiety sufferers aren't. Take note of what you say to yourself. Do you expect life to play by your rules? Do you demand that you should get out of life what you put in? Must life give you your just desserts?

The thing is that life doesn't work like that. Sometimes it gives you bad breaks which you don't deserve. But at other times it will present you with a bouquet which you haven't earned. Some of my patients seemed unable to see the gifts and good fortune that came their way, while focusing entirely on the misfortune and dangers that assailed them.

So give up your search for fairness in life. You'll never find it. Look instead for opportunities. When they present themselves, act on them. Don't assume that, just because things have gone wrong in the past, they will automatically do so in the future. If you flip a coin four times and it comes up tails on each occasion, the chances of it coming up heads next time is exactly 50 per cent. Don't give in to superstition, it's bunkum.

Coping

What you do is more important than how you feel about it. If you are starting to approach the things you fear, don't expect to do so with cool insouciance. You may be a bundle of nerves, but that doesn't matter. Just get it done. What you're after isn't perfection or even calmness; that'll happen later. For now, just look to do what you need to in order to cope with what faces you. Getting started with facing your anxiety and coping with it are the hardest and most important steps. Take that step and the rest will follow.

Start, but don't finish

Tackling anxiety and your avoidance of what you fear is hard. If you find that you aren't doing something which is hard but which you meant to do, it's probably that you were expecting too much of yourself. You know that achieving your objective in one go is going to be horribly difficult, so your brain recoils from it and you find yourself not getting started. So don't try to achieve it all in one go. Just get started. Baby steps. A part-done task is better than a completed one, because it isn't painful and so you're more likely to keep going and to get to your objective in the end. Don't make your life any more uncomfortable than it needs to be.

This goes against what most of us were taught as kids. 'If you start something, finish it.' 'Persevere until it's completed.' 'You don't get to play until you've finished your homework.' All good principles to teach your kids, up to a point. But with the task of dealing with anxiety, all of that needs to be turned on its head. 'Start, but don't finish – yet.' 'Have a go, but if it doesn't go well, don't worry, have another go tomorrow.' 'It'll get done when it's done.' 'Do a bit of homework, then go and play. Come back to your homework later.' These are much better principles for you right now.

I hope that the advice in this chapter helps. Don't worry if you don't make great strides at this stage. I've outlined these ideas so that you can start to work on them while you're waiting for professional help to start. They aren't an alternative to therapy, but a preparation for it. If I'm wrong and carrying out these principles brings your anxiety under control satisfactorily, all the better, but no matter if not. You've made a start and that's a triumph.

7

Psychological treatments

This chapter is a brief introduction to some of the psychological treatments that are available for anxiety states. They all work – there is a wealth of proof for their efficacy. If you haven't yet approached your GP to ask about treatment, please do so. There may be a waiting list for treatment, so the sooner you get on it, the sooner you'll get relief from your anxiety. Stick with it, as any therapy is likely to take time to be effective. Your symptoms may then return after a while, if so you may need more than one spell of therapy. But eventually, if you stick with what you're taught, there is a very good chance that you will be able to conquer your fear permanently.

If you are awaiting the start of your therapy, this is some of what you may expect.

Cognitive-behavioural therapy (CBT)

This is the longest established of the psychological treatments for anxiety that are widely used now. Its starting point is the cognitive triad described by the psychologist Aaron Beck (see Chapter 2). A person suffering from an anxiety disorder has a negative view of herself (powerless, worthless, vulnerable), the world (hostile, dangerous, unpredictable) and the future (full of danger, disasters, pitfalls for the unwary).

CBT is about identifying first the negative thoughts making up this cognitive triad, then the deeply held underlying assumptions which generate these thoughts. Next, these thoughts are challenged in a structured and logical way. Then, behavioural experiments are set up to test out the different ways of viewing your situation. Last, you reflect with your therapist on the results of these experiments and decide on how to alter your thoughts and assumptions based on the evidence you have found. This is a continuous process, as anxiety is tenacious. New negative thoughts pop up which reflect unhelpful underlying assumptions of which you were previously unaware. Each time one is revealed you deal with it in the same structured way. This process is like dealing with a leaky boat. You seal one leak, only for another to appear, then another. Eventually all of the leaks are sealed and the boat can safely sail. It's about persistence. This is the 'cognitive' bit of CBT.

CBT also involves getting good at the strategies I outlined in the last two chapters, particularly relaxation and 'Avoiding avoidance'. That's the 'Behavioural' part of CBT. The principle of *reciprocal inhibition* is that you can't be both anxious and relaxed at the same time. If you get really good at relaxation and then combine a relaxation exercise with whatever makes you anxious, you begin to unravel the vicious cycles of fear of fear and avoidance leading to more fear. The other important principle is of *systematic desensitization*. That is, you draw up a list of feared situations, like rungs on a ladder, with only slightly scary situations at the bottom and the most feared situation at the top. You start at the bottom and, one rung at a time, slowly climb the ladder, all the time combining each rung with your relaxation exercise. If you suffer from GAD (see Chapter 1), you may not have rungs to the ladder as your fear has no focus – you are just anxious all of the time. However, it's still going to be important to identify any thing or situation that you're avoiding. Start to approach it and practise your relaxation exercise as you do so. In any case, you need to be practising your relaxation exercise for at least half an hour every day. I know you haven't got time, but you need to make time. This is probably the most important factor that will determine whether or not your therapy works.

Let's look at an example of how CBT may work in practice. I will again use a case of social anxiety as an example, because it illustrates well the way CBT works, but the same principles apply whatever form of anxiety you suffer from.

Meg is very lacking in confidence. She has a low opinion of herself and considers herself unattractive, stupid and boring. As a result, she avoids social events whenever she can, goes out very little and keeps herself to herself at work. She avoids talking to people, not because she is happy in her own company but because she fears being humiliated if social interactions go wrong. Whenever she does talk to someone, she cringes inside and berates herself for her lack of social skill. She stammers, blushes and often loses her thread of thought, because she is so anxious. And so the vicious cycle of fear of fear and avoidance is set up and Meg becomes increasingly isolated. She longs for a circle of friends and a loving relationship with a steady partner, but these are impossible fantasies for her.

Then Meg starts in CBT, having already learnt and practised a relaxation exercise daily for the several months she was on the waiting list for therapy.

Meg's therapist starts by looking at her fears and the deeply held underlying assumptions which generate them. These can be grouped into six main categories:

1 I'm no good (ugly, stupid, boring).
2 I will always fail.
3 Nobody will like me and everyone will laugh at my blushing, stammering and brain-freezes.
4 I am the most socially unskilled person in the world.
5 I should be better than this.
6 Humiliation is the worst thing that can happen to me and must be avoided.

Some of these assumptions can be worked on straight away. For example, Meg hasn't always failed. In fact, she did well at school and went on to do well at secretarial college, despite getting little encouragement at home and being bullied for much of her time at secondary school. Her parents fought for most of her formative years and her elder brother, who was athletic and popular, teased her for fun whenever the chance arose. Despite witnessing mostly cruelty and abuse at home and at school, Meg's end-of-term reports usually commended her diligence and her kindness.

Is Meg boring? It depends on your perspective. If you're an outgoing, sporty 'jock', then maybe so, as you'll have little in common with Meg. But if your interests are quieter, including classical music, historical novels and the cinema, she certainly isn't boring, as Meg has an encyclopaedic knowledge of these subjects. She assumes that these interests are worthless, but her therapist will challenge this unhelpful value judgement.

Should Meg be better than this? Why? How is it that it's OK and understandable for someone else with a background like hers to be shy and retiring, when it isn't OK for Meg? How come the double standard?

Meg's therapist will spend some time picking through these harmful thoughts and assumptions, gently and methodically challenging them one by one. Even more importantly, Meg will be encouraged to start challenging them herself.

Important though this 'cognitive' work is in attempting to change the way Meg thinks about herself, the world and the future, it can only go so far. At some point it's going to have to be tried out in the real world. Her therapist is then going to set up some 'behavioural experiments'. These won't be too ambitious to start with, as there's no point in Meg being traumatized by being pushed into something that is terrifying for her. So she is asked to draw up a hierarchy of feared situations, with the least scary at the beginning and the most feared at the end:

1 Ask my cousin Sue to go to the local coffee shop with me.
2 Sit with the women from the office at lunch instead of sitting on my own.
3 Go to the pub with my colleagues on Friday after work for Brian's leaving drinks do (for half an hour – make an excuse to leave early).
4 Talk to Jen during the morning coffee break (she's friendly).
5 Talk to my single neighbour Phil when I see him at the gate (he usually leaves for work at the same time I do and he seems really nice).
6 Ask Phil if he'd like to pop down to our local for a drink.

In practice, a real hierarchy of feared situations will probably be much longer than this one, but the one here is for illustration. At this stage, Meg would be as likely to be able to ask Phil out for a drink as to fly to the moon, but that will come later, in its own good time, when Meg has gained confidence from the earlier steps. That's the purpose of the hierarchy. Lots of little steps, no huge leaps. You ascend the mountain by taking thousands of small steps.

So let's take one of these steps, number two, and follow it through. Towards the end of the morning at work, Meg will excuse herself, retire to the loo and practise a relaxation exercise, then go on to the canteen for lunch at 12.35, just after the rest of the office. She will then go to the table where her colleagues are seated and ask if it's OK if she joins them. 'Sure,' says Jen, speaking for the group, which then resumes its discussions around the unfairness of the new work targets and the physical attributes of the young guy who has been taken on as an intern for the summer. Meg mostly doesn't have the confidence to take part in these conversations, except to say that the new targets are making it hard for her to get her work done in time to catch the 6pm train home. Nina laughs and says that's because Meg's typing is too slow. Meg can't think of a witty retort to that and is silent for the rest of the lunch. She then spends the rest of the day beating herself up for not being more talkative, witty or assertive. 'I'm so useless, I can't even hold my own for half an hour at lunch.'

The next day at her CBT session, Meg's therapist goes over the events of the lunch break with her. First, Meg's assumption that it was a disaster is challenged. Meg's perfect standard of how she should have performed is dismantled. It isn't realistic. The truth is that she managed to go and sit with her colleagues for the first time and then to make it through the full half-hour. She even managed to say something, which in the circumstances was a triumph. Realistically, Nina's jibe was only a clumsy attempt at humour, which she's known for, not a real criticism. As it happens, Meg's typing speed is roughly average for the office (they all took a speed test last month). It was a good thing that Meg didn't argue with Nina, as that would have come over as defensive. All in all, a good start. Meg isn't convinced and so her therapist asks her to assess the likelihood of each possible conclusion concerning the exchange with Nina:

- Nina thinks that I'm a lousy typist – 20%.
- Everyone thinks that I'm a lousy typist – 40%.
- Nina was being mean to hurt me – 20%.
- Nina was joking – 20%.

Meg then agrees with her therapist that she'll check with Jen, who she knows is kind, when she next meets her by the coffee machine, which Meg does the next day.

'Hey Jen, you know when I joined you for lunch the other day?'

'Yes, it was nice that you joined us.'

'You remember Nina said I was too slow at typing – does everyone think that?'

'What, of course not. Don't be so sensitive Meg, that's just Nina being Nina. You beat me in the typing speed test, didn't you? Actually, I think you beat Nina too!'

At her next CBT session this interaction is discussed and the probabilities exercise repeated:

- Nina thinks that I'm a lousy typist – 5%.
- Everyone thinks I'm a lousy typist – 0%.
- Nina was being mean to hurt me – 5%.
- Nina was joking – 90%.

So now Meg has a changed conclusion to work with. Her therapist then takes this evidence back to her underlying assumptions, starting with 'I'm no good' and 'I will always fail'. The evidence from these behavioural experiments are compared with her assumptions and Meg is helped to see the inconsistencies. She didn't fail and, apparently, she is a passably good typist.

As you can imagine, there are going to need to be a lot of behavioural experiments, a lot of teasing out of Meg's false assumptions and some nudging along to change them. Successful CBT can take a while and sometimes you may need to come back for another go. Stick at it though. If you are offered only a few sessions and they aren't enough, push for more. If this doesn't work, keep working on this stuff yourself or with a friend or family member, or get one of the online CBT apps. FearFighter and SilverCloud are two such programmes which come highly recommended, but you'll need to access them through a referral by your GP or mental health professional. Catch I is a CBT app for your smartphone or tablet which is free from the App Store. CBT self-help books include *The Anxiety and Phobia Workbook*, by Edmund Bourne. One caution with self-help materials: they can make things worse if you try to carry them out perfectly and if you blame yourself for a lack of progress in the short term. Remember, this isn't a test, it's a process and it may be a slow one, aimed at helping you little by little to change the way you think, feel and live your life. There may be two steps forward and one step back, but persistence usually wins in the end.

There are different varieties of CBT, so don't worry if the treatment you're offered doesn't follow exactly the model I've outlined here. For example, one variant is called cognitive-analytical therapy (CAT). This, as the name suggests, combines CBT with some exploration of the experiences and emotions from earlier in your life which brought you to the place in which you find yourself now. It suits some people, particularly those whose anxiety has very clear origins in early life trauma.

Mindfulness (Mindfulness-Based CBT, MBCBT)

This is an offshoot of CBT, based on the principles of Buddhist and other Eastern philosophies. It was developed by the American scientist Jon Kabat-Zinn, among others. He is the author of *Wherever You Go, There You Are: Mindfulness meditation for everyday life* (Hyperion, 2004), which is highly recommended. He, in turn, followed the earlier work by Eckhart Tolle, the author of the bestseller *The Power of Now*, first released in 1997, but now published by New World Library (2004).

Tolle is an interesting character. He had what seemed a great life, with a great job, wealth, respect and a good relationship, but he was miserable. So much so that he considered suicide. Fortunately, he didn't carry this through but, instead, he thought long and hard about why he was so unhappy. He came to the conclusion that it was because he never really enjoyed all of the trappings of his success, because he was spending so much time either ruminating regretfully about everything he had got wrong and the wrongs that had been done to him or, alternatively, worrying about all that could go wrong in the future. So he came up with a radical solution, which was to give it all up. And I mean give it *all* up. He gave up his job, his girlfriend, his house and his money and went to live as a tramp, begging for food and spending his days meditating. At the end of a year or so he had in his head the book which was to be *The Power of Now* and became a multi-million bestseller, making him wealthy again. Funny how life works like that.

Tolle's message is, therefore, in essence simple: learn how to live in the present and your problems will evaporate. It isn't the stuff that happens to us that causes most of our suffering, but us beating ourselves up for our mistakes, railing against the unfairness of what has happened and fearing the vicissitudes of the future. It's all a myth anyway, because we remember selectively. Those who suffer from anxiety tend to remember events as more negative and traumatic than they would have been rated as by an impartial observer. They also fear all sorts of catastrophes, 99 per cent of which never happen. That's not to say that bad things never happen, but those that do tend to fall out of a clear blue sky. Your worry is a fantasy from which you need to escape. You can do so by being truly present. Do read *The Power of Now*. It's a good read.

While we're on the subject of reading material, *Mindfulness: A practical guide to finding peace in a frantic world* (Mark Williams and Danny Penman, 2011, Hachette Digital) is probably the best material on the subject for the British market. The app Headspace, available for Apple and Android devices and free for the first ten days, is good for those who prefer something they can listen to. It has three 'basic' guided meditations and then a library of topics to choose from including stress, anxiety, cravings and others. The meditations last from three minutes to over 20 minutes, so as you become more expert, depending on how much time you have, you can increase the time you meditate. I'm told that the app Calm is also very good and is free to try out, so it may be worth checking out, though I haven't used it myself.

I am simplifying somewhat, but mindfulness has, for me, two main principles. The first is being really *present* in the moment, which I've already discussed. The other is to *stop fighting*.

That means stop fighting the past, the future, unfairness, your symptoms, your feelings and emotions, your perceived inadequacies, everything. Just experience *being. Don't just do something, sit there*. Remember what I said earlier about the worst part of anxiety being the *fear of fear*? A mindfulness therapist will encourage you to accept and experience your anxiety, rather than fight with it. Anxiety is perverse in that way, like a dog with someone who doesn't like dogs: try to push it away and it will only increase its interest and bother you more; accept it, even welcome it and it will leave you alone. Rather than trying to ignore and avoid the physical symptoms of anxiety and the racing thoughts which you are suffering, be aware of them and experience them for what they are: normal, harmless and transient experiences. Like the flock of birds I brought up in the last chapter. Don't judge your symptoms and thoughts or make conclusions from them, just experience them.

I had a mindfulness test for my patients. As you entered the building, there was a flower bed by the main entrance. What colour were the flowers? Most couldn't answer this question because they were so busy thinking about the upcoming appointment or the troubles they had been suffering in the period leading up to it. But the past is gone. The appointment will arrive soon enough and there will be plenty of time to go through your problems when it arrives. What is available to you in the moments when you are walking towards the front entrance is a flower bed. Experience it in the moment. It's the only thing at that moment that is real.

Mindfulness, while being simple in principle, is tricky to carry off, so you may need some help with it. While many individual therapists incorporate it into their sessions, mindfulness is often taught in groups. If you are offered to join such a group, take it up. There is very good evidence for the method's efficacy. You won't be required to interact much with the other group members, unless you choose to, so if you're socially anxious, you don't need to fear being exposed to difficult social demands.

Acceptance and commitment therapy (ACT)

This is a form of MBCBT that is gaining increasing popularity. The focus is there in the name. Accept your symptoms and, even more, your limitations and difficulties. Don't avoid them or try to escape from them. Let your feelings be. Allow yourself not to be good at everything. Observe your weaknesses rather than judging yourself for them and acknowledge your strengths. Forget the 'why?' – accept the reality and work with what you have.

ACT can be a different acronym:	Accept your reactions and stay present Choose a valued direction Take action

While your feelings and your symptoms are what they are, you can control how you react to them. This is where the commitment comes in. You'll agree with your therapist on a changed course of action and then commit to it, however it makes you feel, while at the same time acknowledging and experiencing the feelings.

Feelings are tough, particularly when they're caused by another person. 'Sticks and stones may break my bones' … but words hurt a lot worse. That's why it is helpful to have a therapist to help you to stay on course while not avoiding your feelings.

ACT works well for most anxiety disorders. If you want to read more, go to *Get Out of Your Mind and Into Your Life: The New Acceptance and Commitment Therapy* by Steven Hayes and Spencer Smith (New Harbinger Publications, 2005).

Exploratory therapies for anxiety

The majority of the psychological therapy carried out under the NHS in the UK is based on CBT (with more or less emphasis on the cognitive element, depending on the problem being treated) and Mindfulness. For most people suffering with anxiety disorders, focusing on the here and now and enabling a change in thinking and behaviour seems to be of at least as much benefit as exploring the past origins of your fear. It's also a lot quicker, with CBT typically involving 6 to 20 sessions, while exploratory psychotherapy may need sessions once or more a week for months to years.

Gaining insight into how you got to the point you're at doesn't necessarily translate into relief of symptoms. However, developing insight is only one element of exploratory (psycho-dynamic) psychotherapy (EP). Probably more important is the relationship you develop with your therapist. In EP, your therapist will encourage you to look at the feelings you experience within the sessions as well as those you come in with. Typically, over time you will develop feelings about the sessions and about your therapist which mirror feelings and experiences you have had with pivotal people earlier in your life. This is called 'trans-ference'. Many exploratory therapists consider that working through transference is the most powerful way of repairing damage done by problems in harmful relationships in your past, particularly in childhood.

From this brief, simplified description of how EP works, you can see that some people are likely to get benefits from this kind of therapy, which they might not gain from therapies focused on present thinking and behaviours. If, for example, you have suffered bullying at home and at school throughout childhood, you may find that one relationship after another in adulthood is torpedoed by your anxiety, lack of trust and avoidance of intimacy. You just can't let go. These feelings are likely to come into the therapy too, with you having difficulty trusting your therapist. By working through the fear that is holding you back within the safety of the therapeutic relationship, you may learn how to trust in other settings too. This is just an example, but it illustrates why some people benefit from some exploration beyond the CBT model.

In practice, years of EP isn't practical for most people and it isn't usually available under the NHS. However, short-Term focal psychotherapy may successfully resolve a single issue underpinning your anxiety in only a few sessions. As the name suggests, it is a short form of therapy focusing specifically on the issue at hand, rather than involving an exploration of your whole life. CAT (see above under CBT) also tends to be quicker than full-blown EP, so is sometimes available under the NHS.

Alternative therapies

I'm not going to go into the various 'alternative' psychological treatments here, as they really aren't my thing. My training is in the scientific practice of medicine, resting mainly on the evidence of research, though I'm also informed by my own and colleagues' clinical experience and the experiences of my patients. Alternative therapies, in contrast, aren't a science but an art and so don't have a large weight of research evidence to back them up. I'm not saying that an alternative therapy won't work for you, it might. But asking me about it is like asking a painter and decorator about a Leonardo da Vinci painting. He may be able to tell about the paint used, but that'll be about it. But look, if you believe in it and it works for you, go for it. Benefits you gain from anything is valid evidence, for you. Don't though be led by your friend Bill, who says the best treatment for anxiety is to sit for five hours a day under a piece of moon rock (which he's happy to sell you) and who tells you to avoid doctors. I don't get my legal advice from my butcher. Go and see your GP.

There is some research evidence for hypnosis and for acupuncture to treat anxiety disorders, but I don't think the weight of it compares with that for the therapies I've outlined here. Transcendental meditation does have an evidence base, which is not surprising as it has a lot in common with the practice of mindfulness.

Again, I'm not going to discuss religion here, as it's not what this book is about. I would just say this though. Many of my patients appear to have been helped immeasurably by their religion. If you are religious, seek help there, but don't let anyone tell you that your anxiety is a result of sin, or you not praying enough. Some of my most anxious patients have also been the most devout.

If the therapy you need isn't immediately available through your local healthcare provider, first push a bit. The squeaky wheel gets the oil, as they say. If you have severe and enduring problems with anxiety which are blighting your life, you are entitled to effective treatment. Push for it if you need to. If you still come up empty handed and have access to funds, consider seeking psychological therapy privately. Get advice from your GP on what treatment to seek and from whom. GPs know who the best therapists are and there are some therapists and counsellors who are not worth your hard-earned cash. If you have private medical insurance, you may need to be referred to a psychiatrist (a doctor specializing in mental health) to diagnose and oversee your treatment. In my view, it's no bad thing to be seen by a psychiatrist anyway since self-diagnosis isn't always reliable, the first model of therapy doesn't always prove effective and, sometimes, the addition of medication is necessary for the psychological therapy to work.

8

Medications for anxiety disorders

Very few subjects attract more heated debate than the role of drug treatments in anxiety. Everyone seems to have a view which they are more than happy to impose on you. The general rule that the strength of a person's opinion is inversely proportional to their knowledge and wisdom holds here. In other words, be sceptical about sensational headlines which you see in the press from time to time about the efficacy or otherwise of medications for treatment of anxiety. They aren't placebos, but they aren't panaceas either.

A lot of the more sensational pronouncements about medications in psychiatry have been about antidepressants in depression, but the same advocates also pronounce upon these and other drugs in anxiety, so I'll touch on the controversy here. I'd love to go on at length about 'fake news' dressed up as research in this area, but I suspect that I'd bore you into a stupor. Suffice it to say that diagnosis, thresholds of significance and the strength of the placebo effect all make research difficult to interpret. When is anxiety a diagnosis and when just an emotion? How severe does it need to be to have you included in a drug trial? Does the medication tested only work for some types of anxiety disorder, in which case will it fail to demonstrate its efficacy in a study including everyone suffering from anxiety? How much reduction in anxiety is significant? How strong is the placebo effect? I'll answer three of these questions. Medications are helpful mainly for more severe anxiety disorders and are much more effective for some disorders than for others. A recent article by Professor Gordon Parker in the *British Journal of Psychiatry* pointed out that if you lumped together all people with 'severe breathlessness' as if this were a diagnosis, you'd end up giving many of them ineffective treatment, since drugs effective for bronchitis won't work for asthma and some drugs effective for breathlessness caused by anxiety may make asthma worse. The same problem occurs if you group together in a research study people suffering from different types of anxiety disorder.

The placebo effect is very strong, as is the effect of being interviewed by a doctor in a research study. In a study looking at tranquillizer withdrawal which I carried out some years ago, we had two initial interviews with the patients included in the trial built into the protocol. They were two weeks apart before the withdrawal process started. These interviews were principally to measure baseline levels of anxiety in the subjects. The researchers were instructed not to do any therapy in these sessions, but just to administer the various rating scales and other measures. In practice though, the researchers, being caring people, chatted supportively with the subjects, asking them how they were doing, sympathizing with their complaints, asking after their pets and such like. As a result of nothing more than these 'chats', the average level of anxiety of the group halved during the run-in period. It seems that non-specific factors like supportive human contact have a very potent effect on anxiety.

So research is difficult to interpret. But I try to do so, and this chapter summarizes my conclusions. Here's a summary before we begin: if psychological methods work well for you, don't bother with medications but, if your anxiety disorder is so severe that it stops you from being able to engage effectively with therapy, you may benefit greatly from appropriate medication. You can't do therapy if you're in a state of blind terror. Taking the edge off with medication may allow you to go from terrified to anxious but able to think and act effectively. The aim isn't to abolish your anxiety with medication, as it'll only come back when you come off the drug, but to reduce it sufficiently for you to be able to do what you need to for the therapy to deal with your anxiety long term. While a few people need to remain on medications indefinitely, most can slowly withdraw from them once the psychological therapy has worked.

Here are the types of medications most often used to treat anxiety disorders.

SSRI antidepressants

These drugs (serotonin-specific reuptake inhibitors, SSRIs) work, as their name suggests, principally on the neurotransmitter serotonin. They include fluoxetine (Prozac), paroxetine (Seroxat), citalopram (Cipramil), escitalopram (Cipralex) and fluvoxamine (Faverin). Buspirone (Buspar), marketed primarily as an anti-anxiety drug, works similarly. The SSRIs are generally regarded as the first line of medication treatment for anxiety disorders.

The most important thing to be aware of with SSRI medications is that they tend to make you feel worse to begin with, maybe for up to two weeks. Persevere if you can, because this initial side effect usually wears off and the beneficial effect can take four to six weeks to kick in. If you feel really awful, you should stop taking the drug, but then see your GP as soon as possible, as there may well be another drug which you'll find easier to start. Once established on an SSRI, take it every day until your doctor advises you to stop taking it. They don't work if you miss doses.

Because the anxiety-reducing effect is delayed, SSRIs have very little addictive potential. Any drug that works immediately carries this risk because of the power of conditioning (see Chapter 2). Reduction of anxiety paired with taking a pill creates a strong pull towards continuing to take that pill (craving). As no such immediate pairing occurs with SSRIs, there is little or no craving to take it. Having said all this, you should not stop an SSRI suddenly after having taken it regularly for a while, as you may suffer withdrawal symptoms if you do. If you come off by tapering down the drug slowly over a few weeks, you shouldn't have a problem.

SSRIs can be very helpful for people suffering from a severe anxiety disorder. Essentially, they buy you time, reducing your anxiety for long enough for you to be able to engage successfully with the psychological therapy that will provide the permanent solution to your symptoms. Because they seem to be safe to take long term, there is no urgency to come off them, although it's probably a good idea to do so eventually if you can and unless your doctor advises against it.

There are some cautions on using SSRIs, as there are with all drugs. Because they can cause initial worsening of symptoms, anyone who has had suicidal thoughts should think twice about starting one unless they have a fairly constant source of support available. If you have epilepsy, heart, liver or kidney problems, glaucoma or diabetes, make sure the doctor prescribing the drug is aware of these. They may interact with other drugs you're taking so, again, make sure your doctor has a list of all your medications, including over-the-counter products like aspirin. SSRIs may cause sexual dysfunction in some, in particular difficulty reaching orgasm. This resolves once you come off the drug, though more persistent sexual difficulties can arise if you become anxious about sex or if you lose interest in it after a long time on an SSRI.

Other antidepressants

Most of the antidepressant drugs which have been around for longer than the SSRIs also reduce anxiety. Examples are the Tricyclics such as amitriptyline, imipramine, clomipramine and dosulepin (these don't have trade names any more as the original manufacturers have mostly stopped producing them). Related and slightly newer drugs include trazodone (Molipaxin) and lofepramine (Gamanil). Tricyclics are less used than SSRIs nowadays as they tend to have more side effects and are dangerous in overdosage. They can be useful though for those who don't get on with SSRIs or who need help sleeping. They are mostly quite sedative and are an option for those who need a hypnotic with little or no addictive potential.

The MAOIs (monoamine oxidase inhibitors) are even older than the tricyclics, having been around for over 60 years. Examples are phenelzine (Nardil) and tranylcypromine. They are also little used, because of a number of inconvenient side effects and dietary restrictions. It is dangerous to eat cheese, yeast products or to consume anything fermented, particularly red wine, when taking an MAOI. There are also a number of interactions with other medicines which need to be avoided. There is a newer, related drug, moclobemide (Manerix), which avoids some of these problems, although there is some doubt over whether it works as well as the older drugs. MAOIs are thought by some to be particularly effective in treating panic disorder, phobic anxiety and health anxiety disorder, although I didn't use them routinely in my practice owing to the difficulties involved in taking them which I've mentioned.

Newer antidepressants are probably also effective in treating anxiety disorders. They include venlafaxine (Efexor), which is a powerful antidepressant, but may be more risky in those suffering with heart disease and possibly more difficult to get off than the SSRIs for some. Mirtazapine is quite sedative, so may be good for those with insomnia, and tends to cause less sexual dysfunction than the SSRIs, but it can sometimes cause a ferocious increase in appetite resulting in troublesome weight gain. Once in a blue moon, it may cause a potentially dangerous side effect in which some types of white blood cells stop being produced by the body (agranulocytosis). The symptoms of this rare complication are just like flu. If you develop a fever and feel rotten soon after starting mirtazapine, stop taking it and see your GP as soon as possible. It is reversible, but it needs to be caught quickly. The chances are that you've picked up a virus, but it's better not to risk it until a simple blood test rules out agranulocytosis.

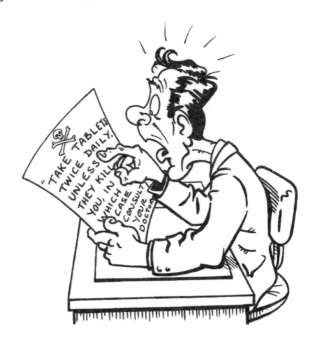

This is a whistle-stop tour of the antidepressant drugs and includes only a smattering of relevant information about them. Read the patient information leaflet (PIL) which comes with your tablets, though do take it with a pinch of salt. Manufacturers have to include every side effect that has ever been reported, even once, anywhere in the world with their drug. If you read the PIL for paracetamol, the side effect list would end with 'syncope, coma and death', which is terrifying, but most of us use it quite safely whenever we get a headache. If you're worried about any side effect, go and talk to your GP about it.

Benzodiazepines

When I first started practising in psychiatry, these tranquillizers, which work on the GABA system in the brain (see Chapter 2), were handed out at the drop of a hat for almost any complaint, or just for unhappiness. Then reports started emerging of people becoming dependent on the drugs and suffering withdrawal symptoms when they tried to stop them. As so often happens, the medical profession and the public we serve swung the other way. Change usually happens by revolution rather than by a slow and sensible shift, and the history of tranquillizer use is no exception. Diazepam (Valium), chlordiazepoxide (Librium), lorazepam (Ativan) and alprazolam (Xanax) were demonized as dangerously addictive drugs to be avoided at all costs. That, in my opinion, is a shame since, as usual, the truth lies in the middle.

Benzodiazepine tranquillizers are potentially addictive, but not very strongly so. Alcohol is too, but most of us use it quite happily and without problems. It's a bad idea for someone with a history of, or propensity for, addiction to drink alcohol, and equally unwise for them to use tranquillizers. The available research shows that even most people who take benzodiazepines regularly don't escalate their dose. Most regular users who withdraw in a slow stepwise manner manage to do so without severe withdrawal symptoms.

The problem with these drugs is that *they work, immediately.* This is in contrast to the SSRIs, which take days or weeks to work. If you've been suffering from severe anxiety which is alleviated straight away by taking a pill, there will be a strong pull (psychological dependence) towards continuing to take it, which doesn't occur with a pill that has a delayed effect. That is, unless you use the pill only to buy you time, to reduce your anxiety short term just enough for you to do the work in therapy that you need to do in order to achieve the long-term result you're looking for.

So benzodiazepines are a short-term solution for those who struggle with the first two weeks on an SSRI or for whom those drugs prove ineffective. They are also potentially useful to get you started in therapy, if this is proving an impossible hurdle for you. Say you've been struggling with phobic anxiety and drawn up your hierarchy of feared situations, but just can't get started with the first rung on the ladder because your anxiety is too severe. Using a tranquillizer as a one-off may get you started as, once you've managed the first rung, the others tend to be easier. Be careful with this though. It's not a solution to take diazepam every time you do something you fear. Only use it over the short term (a few days max) or occasionally. Specific situational fears, such as fear of flying, are another possible occasional use. Make sure to test out the drug before you fly though. People's responses to benzodiazepines are very variable. If you happen to be unusually sensitive to them and you take one for the first time just before getting to the airport, there is a risk that you may turn up appearing drunk and be refused your seat on the plane. Try one for the first time when it doesn't matter, such as on a quiet Sunday at home, so that you can assess the drug's effect on you and the dose that is effective. Oh, and don't drive under the influence of a tranquillizer.

Intuitively, I feel that benzodiazepines should be particularly helpful for panic attacks, as such episodes need a fast-acting remedy and only happen intermittently. Unfortunately, some research shows that these drugs don't work well for panic disorder.

There are other benzodiazepines which have been used as sleeping tablets (temazepam, for example), but these have largely been superseded by the related 'Z-drugs': zopiclone, zolpidem and zaleplon. While working on the same chemical system as benzodiazepines, these drugs have a more subtle mode of action, having a stronger effect on promoting sleep than on reducing anxiety. While not being strongly addictive, they need to be used with the same caution as benzodiazepine tranquillizers.

Anti-epileptics

Most drugs used to treat epilepsy have a tranquillizing effect. They aren't widely used yet to treat anxiety disorders, but I expect them to be more often prescribed in the future, owing to their safety (in those not suffering from kidney disease or heart failure) and low addictive potential. The anti-epileptic drug most widely prescribed for anxiety disorders is pregabalin (Lyrica). If you need an anti-anxiety medication for longer-term use, but don't get on with SSRIs or other antidepressants, then pregabalin may be an option. It is expensive at the time of writing and so some GPs are reluctant to prescribe it.

Beta blockers

Beta blockers are, essentially, anti-adrenaline drugs, though only combating the effects of this hormone on the body, not the brain. They can be helpful for those afflicted by the physical symptoms of anxiety, particularly on performance. I used to play the violin and suffered a troubling tremor of my hand when I performed in public, causing the bow to bounce on the strings. The more it happened, the more conscious I became that everyone in the audience could tell how anxious I was and the more embarrassed I became, feeding into a vicious cycle. Propranolol, a beta blocker with wide-ranging effects, was helpful in reducing my tremor, although it did tend to worsen my mild asthma. It should not be taken by anyone suffering from severe asthma.

Beta blockers may help some people whose social phobia is driven by self-consciousness over blushing, tremors or other physical effects of anxiety, although research studies in this area have yielded rather disappointing results. One would expect them to be helpful in combating the physical symptoms of panic attacks, but there is little research that confirms this. They may be worth a try if your main concern is other people seeing manifestations of your anxiety, such as if you have to give presentations at work. As with all medications used occasionally to get through specific situations, don't try it for the first time when it really matters. Only take these drugs under the advice of your doctor.

Antipsychotic medicines

These drugs, primarily used to treat psychotic illnesses such as schizophrenia, are also called 'major tranquillizers' and so would be expected to help people suffering from anxiety. In practice, they aren't usually as effective as the drugs I have listed above. They are often prescribed because of fear about the dependence risk with benzodiazepines, but the validity of this indication is dubious as antipsychotics pose risks of their own in long-term use (in particular, the development of abnormal involuntary movements (tardive dyskinesia)). If they work for you, all well and good, but don't use them long term unless you've been advised to do so by your doctor.

Herbal remedies

The fact that herbal remedies and other 'alternative' treatments are so popular is, in my view, owing to a basic misconception, namely that 'natural' is better and safer. You disagree? OK, then you take the hemlock while I stick to Coca-Cola. Herbal remedies often contain a variety of substances, many of which have never been tested for safety or efficacy. They don't have to go through the rigorous testing required of pharmaceutical compounds. They have just as many interactions with other medications as do medically prescribed drugs. Because a substance is naturally occurring doesn't make it safe. While it is an important drug in bipolar disorder, the naturally occurring salt lithium carbonate is the most potentially toxic drug that I prescribed.

This isn't to say that herbal remedies can never work. Hey, if an extract of the dung of the Atlas beetle works for you, use it, presuming you are happy that it's safe. I have nothing against placebos, which can have potent beneficial effects in those who believe in them. Tell your GP that you're taking it though and bring anything that says what it contains with you, in case your remedy includes active compounds that may interact with your other medicines.

There is little good evidence for the efficacy of most herbal remedies, although there is a smattering of evidence that hawthorn, chamomile, lemon balm and passion flower may be more active than placebo in anxiety. There is stronger evidence for the efficacy of kava, but it has been associated with liver damage, sometimes severe, and so it is not prescribed in the UK.

Opiates, alcohol and other no-nos

Opiate analgesics, that is drugs acting on the same receptors in the body as opium, morphine and heroin, have a strong anti-anxiety effect, but please don't ever use them as tranquillizers. Codeine is an opiate, albeit a fairly weak one. All opiates produce tolerance fairly rapidly if used regularly. That is, they lose their effect leading to rapid dosage escalation. They have severe withdrawal effects and produce strong craving. That is, they are highly addictive. If you are concerned that your use of opiate painkillers prescribed in the aftermath of an operation is increasing, tell your GP sooner rather than later. There are other painkillers that don't have the risks of opiates and which won't ratchet up your anxiety when you come off them.

Alcohol is a tranquillizer, but a very bad one. In my view, if a manufacturer were to apply for a licence for alcohol as a new drug today, they would be turned down flat, owing to its many side effects, tolerance, withdrawal effects, addictive potential and harmful effects on various parts of the body in regular, heavy use. Don't use it to deal with anxiety. There are much better drugs available, so go and talk to your GP about what you need.

In summary, there are a number of effective medicines available to treat anxiety disorders. Use them if you need to in order to be able to engage effectively with psychological therapy, to buy you time while you find the long-term solution to your fear.

9

Treatment of specific anxiety disorders

Most anxiety disorders respond to most of the measures and treatments that I've listed in the last two chapters. Whatever the type and severity of your anxiety, you are going to need to make changes in your life and learn new skills to combat your fear. If your anxiety is severe and enduring, you're very likely to need some psychological therapy and, if you struggle with this, you'll need some medication in the short to medium term. But there are some differences between the various types of anxiety disorder in terms of what works best, and I'll touch on these here.

Generalized anxiety disorder (GAD)

As I explained in Chapter 1, the problem here is constant over-arousal. You run too hot all the time and adrenaline is driving this. An anti-adrenaline drug (beta blocker) will combat the physical effects of adrenaline, but not the over-heated central nervous system and the fear that caused the release of adrenaline in the first place. Benzodiazepines such as diazepam will calm you down and relax your muscles, which have been in a state of constant tension. The trouble is that, as I explained in Chapter 8, these drugs are potentially addictive in long-term use and GAD is a long-term condition.

SSRI and tricyclic antidepressants don't carry the same risk of dependence as the benzodiazepines and so can be used for longer. Unfortunately, the weight of evidence for their efficacy isn't as strong for GAD as it is for panic disorder (PD). The first two weeks on an SSRI may be difficult and a benzodiazepine may need to be added on an as-required basis during this period. Young people (under 30) seem to be at greater risk of developing suicidal thoughts in this initial period on SSRIs, so it's important to be aware of this and for support to be available.

Anti-epileptic drugs such as pregabalin have very low addictive potential, but tend to be sedative. While being a bit drowsy may be OK in the short term, it is far from ideal if you need the drug for longer.

There is very good evidence that CBT, mindfulness and ACT are effective in treating GAD, and their effects, unlike those of medication, extend into the long term beyond the end of therapy. Having said this, GAD does have a habit of coming back when life turns hostile, so you may need more than one spell of therapy. Having a good CBT-based self-help book or mindfulness app (see Chapter 7) is a good idea, as you may need to return to it from time to time when life becomes complicated. In any case, practising a shortened version of your relaxation exercise or a mindfulness exercise is something I would recommend you do daily for life.

In order to escape from your fear, you're going to need to change the whole way you run your life and the assumptions which you have operated under up until now. Life is not about controlling, achieving or judging, it's about experiencing and continually learning. It's about developing compassion, particularly for yourself, and letting yourself make mistakes. It's about letting life *be* on its own terms, not yours. You can be free of anxiety, but it may be a long haul. One rule that mustn't be broken though: you aren't allowed to criticize yourself if your efforts don't lead to perfect resolution of your anxiety. No judgements, just stick with it.

The bottom line is you should start by making the changes and developing the skills which I set out in Chapters 5 and 6, get referred for some specific therapy through your GP if your GAD is severe and enduring, and only take medication if you need it to allow you to engage effectively in therapy. While antidepressants are safe in long-term use, many people are able slowly to come off them after effective therapy.

Panic disorder (PD)

Just as it is surprising that there isn't stronger evidence that SSRIs are effective in GAD, it is equally so that benzodiazepines don't show up well in research into remedies for PD. They ought to work, as panic attacks are sudden and you'd think that something like diazepam or the even-faster acting lorazepam would be ideal. It's possible that the GABA receptors (see Chapter 2) which benzodiazepines work on get switched off in PD. It may also be that the speed with which panic attacks happen is just too fast for anything to work in time and the vicious cycle of 'fear – physical symptoms – more fear' is too powerful for any chemical to combat it once it's established. That may be why SSRIs and tricyclic antidepressants seem to work better, as they are established in your system before the next panic attack arrives. It's also worth noting that people who take benzodiazepines for PD are more likely to get addicted to them than those who take them for GAD. In any case, SSRIs are the drugs most used for this condition. Some psychiatrists also prescribe pregabalin or beta blockers for PD sufferers who don't get on with antidepressant drugs, although, again, surprisingly it seems that beta blockers often don't work very well.

CBT, mindfulness and ACT all work well for PD. You may need some medication in the early stages to be able to engage well in the therapy. Most important of all, practise a relaxation exercise every day, come rain or shine. It won't work to begin with, but that's not the point. Like any skill, relaxation has to be learnt through repeated practice so that it becomes automatic and can be switched on like a light when you need it. The hardest time to engage in relaxation is when it's needed, particularly when a panic attack is coming on. To begin with, you're doing it to learn it, so don't expect it to work in the heat of battle at first. That may take months of doing it daily, but persevere because it will be worth it in the end.

A personal anecdote which I touched on earlier: I did a relaxation exercise every day of my life for over two years. This was because I suffered a panic attack in my first viva voce exam at medical school. I was being grilled by a fierce examiner on 'ten causes of renal failure in order of frequency'. My mind went blank and as he glared at me over his half-rim specs, I went into full panic and had to leave the room. The medical school was quite understanding and let me retake the exam a year later, but it meant I had to learn how to deal with panic attacks within this time. It took me about three months for the exercise to be of any use at all, nine months or so for it to be effective in anxiety-provoking situations (I got through the exam) and over two years to get to the point I'm at now. I can now switch on relaxation in a matter of seconds when I need it, without doing the full exercise. It's changed my life. I'm told I was a bit slow, as most people get to each of these stages quite a lot faster than I did, but who cares. I got there in the end.

Try to limit your avoidance. If you avoid everything that you feel might bring on an attack, you'll build up a growing list of phobias. Better to get the occasional attack. They pass with time and they don't harm you, even though it feels like they will while you're having them. That doesn't mean that you have to persecute yourself with constant triggers for panic attacks, but it does mean a consistent and systematic approach to them (see Chapter 7, and the section on CBT and systematic desensitization).

Phobic anxiety disorder (PAD)

I think I can be fairly categorical here. The main treatment, the one which everyone suffering from a specific phobia severe enough to interfere with their life needs, is behavioural therapy (BT). By all means include some of the 'C' (cognitive) elements of CBT as well, but the sine qua non is graded exposure to the feared object or situation combined with relaxation (systematic desensitization and reciprocal inhibition – see Chapter 7). The keys here are careful preparation, learning an effective relaxation exercise and drawing up a detailed hierarchy of feared situations with as many rungs as possible to the ladder. No step should be attempted until the previous step has been achieved and can be repeated without too much difficulty. No step should be a giant leap, but only a little more challenging than the one before. You climb the mountain not in ten giant strides, but in a thousand small steps. OK, I'm being metaphorical there; you don't need a thousand steps in your systematic desensitization hierarchy, but you do need enough that no step is too daunting. Nothing should be terrifying or traumatic, but it should be challenging enough to make you a bit anxious, so that your relaxation technique has something to work on. Keep moving forward, slowly but steadily and with persistence. As I've said before, you may need a therapist to help you with this. Get one through your GP. If you don't have a therapist, co-opt a wise friend with whom you can share what you're doing and your progress at it. You may need to get them to read this book, or at least this chapter and Chapter 7, so they know the rationale for your efforts.

In the past, some therapists used 'flooding', that is, leaving you with your most anxiety-provoking situation until your anxiety subsides. So a person with a phobia of spiders is locked in a room full of spiders. Their anxiety rises, peaks and eventually falls as they habituate to their arachnid companions. Once the fear has been faced and overcome, exposure to the same phobic object (in this case spiders) in the future fails to produce the same fear response, as the fear-of-fear vicious cycle has been broken. If you're really impatient or in need of a quick fix, a psychologist may suggest flooding, but I wouldn't recommend it. There's no need for heroism here, just for persistence.

Medication has limited value in treatment of specific phobias. The only time it's worth using anti-anxiety tablets is if you reach a block where you can't get any further or even get started without some temporary help. In this case, short-term help with a few days of a benzodiazepine might get you started. Be careful though; it will be very tempting to continue a tranquillizer if it eliminates your anxiety, but you'll be storing up problems for the future if you do. An alternative, if it's necessary, may be to start an SSRI antidepressant a few weeks before you start the process of BT. Only do this if you can't work through your hierarchy of feared situations without chemical help. Once you are able to, after discussion with your treating doctor, slowly withdraw the medication over a few weeks.

Agoraphobia (AP)

This condition is a phobia and so everything which I've written about PAD applies. But it also has a big overlap with PD. What maintains AP is that whenever you go beyond your comfort zone you suffer a panic attack, which is traumatic and increases your fear and avoidance. The first key, even more than with PAD or PD, is the drawing up of a hierarchy with as many steps of the smallest size as possible. The second is persistence. Keep going, even if you suffer occasional reverses along the way and even if your progress seems painfully slow. The third (I know I'm getting boring, but it really is crucial) is to get good at a relaxation exercise; practise, practise and keep practising.

Say you have become housebound because of panic attacks whenever you get beyond the front door. The first rung on the ladder may be just imagining going out onto the front step. Make sure to combine this imagining with a relaxation exercise. Repeat regularly, maybe once a day or more if you can, until you're able to do this without inducing severe anxiety or panic. Then move on to the second rung, which may be opening the back door one inch and peeking outside for ten seconds. Don't open the door wide just yet and don't be tempted to accelerate the process by going outside. Stick to your prepared hierarchy, taking each planned step (rung of the ladder) in turn. Ideally, the pace of climbing the ladder should seem absurdly slow and the rungs so small that it seems silly. Absurd and silly are the opposites of scary. Whatever you do, don't be heroic. No 'Oh, I'm fed up with this, I'll just take a train to London and spend the day on Oxford Street'. You'll have a nasty panic attack on the platform of the station before you've even started and will find your progress has gone into reverse. Slow and steady are best. My guess is that getting beyond the front gate for ten seconds is probably about ten rungs up the ladder and two or three months at least down the line. Getting to Oxford Street, when it happens, will be only a tiny step beyond what you've already achieved and is probably a couple of years or more in the future.

Seek out support, both from a professional and from a friend or family member who can accompany you in your early forays beyond your comfort zone. If you need medication in the early days to get you started on your hierarchy of fears, use it. I've mentioned that benzodiazepines don't seem to work too well in PD but, if you find you need one to make the first steps and your treating doctor agrees, then use it. Talk to your GP or mental health professional about this. An SSRI may well help you make faster progress too.

CBT (particularly the behavioural part), mindfulness and ACT all work well for AP. If you can't access one-to-one therapy immediately, consider getting online help. I'm not going to suggest a specific online programme here, as it depends on the nature of your difficulties but if, for example, you're on a long waiting list for CBT, call or write to the Psychology Department to which you've been referred and ask their advice about appropriate online resources to help you while you wait.

Social anxiety disorder (SAD)

Phobia of social interaction is the most tricky phobia to treat, but it can be done. It needs time, patience, perseverance and support, both from friends and family on the one hand and from a therapist on the other. It's worth it, as effective treatment can change your life for the better immeasurably.

Like other forms of anxiety, medication may be useful to enable you effectively to engage with the therapy. Benzodiazepines for a day or two may get you started or over what feels like an insuperable hurdle, but don't rely on them long term. SSRIs can be taken for as long as is needed but, once your therapy is complete and you are able to engage in contact with others, you will probably be able slowly to withdraw from your medication. MAOIs (see Chapter 8) are difficult drugs to take, with a lot of restrictions on what you can eat and drink and as many interactions with other medicines, but they do seem to be particularly effective in SAD. Beta blockers may help those who are handicapped by blushing or any other physical manifestation of their anxiety – a drug which stops adrenaline acting on the body can interrupt the 'fear of fear' cycle. If you know that your fear is likely to be less visible to others, you are likely to fear it less. Beta blockers may help with that.

But it is the work done in therapy sessions and between the sessions which yields lasting results. Take it slowly, but steadily. Don't give up. Try to judge yourself less. How you perform in a social situation matters less than whether or not you engage in it. If you meet with a group of acquaintances, and excuse yourself after 20 minutes and leave, that is a success, not a failure. What matters is doing more than you did before. You're not going to do it well, not yet. The main barrier to you overcoming your fear and avoidance of situations isn't your lack of skill or the judgements of others, it's *you* and your unfair criticism of yourself and your social performance. Please, if you take nothing else away from this book, get comfortable with having a go and doing it badly. *The result doesn't matter, it's having a go that counts.* Overcome yourself and your tendency to harsh self-judgement and you'll overcome your SAD. Take each experience you have back to your therapist, who will help you to put it in perspective and to keep going.

Therapy for SAD is usually based on the CBT model, although there is some evidence that short-term exploratory psycho-therapy can also be effective for some.

Exploratory psychotherapy is likely to look at the experiences which led to your fear of social situations and help you to reframe them. I remember an occasion during my time in boarding school when I was alone in the students' common room with the coolest guy in my year. I did something which made him giggle, so I said, 'Don't laugh, it might make your face split.' Not a very funny joke, I know. He shot me a scowl and snarled, 'Cantopher, you can't make me laugh, you're a walking morgue.' That hurt and it affected my confidence for some time, but in due course I reframed it. Looking back, I see that this verbal attack was about him, not me. He was an unhappy kid who needed to be seen as cool and lashed out at others to make him feel better about himself. It's not that I'm the funniest guy around, but I'm me and some people find me OK. Most importantly, I see myself as OK. I got there on my own, with help from my wife and friends, but an exploratory therapist may enable you to look at experiences in your life that have affected you, to work through the hurt and to see them, and so yourself, differently. If this story touches a nerve for you and if significant figures from your past have done and said things that led to your fear of people, you may benefit from exploratory psychotherapy.

If you feel that the past is best left behind and that solutions come from looking forward with a different outlook and more effective strategies, you are sharing a view held by the majority of psychologists. Working with a CBT therapist or psychologist is likely to involve some education about your disorder. They may work with you on social skills, like how to engage in a conversation with someone you meet for the first time. This may involve some use of video to give you feedback on what does and doesn't work well, if you're comfortable with this. Some exercises may be designed to show how focusing on yourself and the impression you are making on others gets in the way of effective functioning and makes you feel worse, as do safety-seeking behaviours (such as saying nothing) and avoidance (such as staying at home). Your therapist will help you to focus more on what is happening, rather than on how you are coming across. They will dig beyond your unhelpful thoughts to the deeply held underlying beliefs which drive them (such as 'I'm no good', 'I'll be humiliated', 'I have to be perfect', 'I'm only as good as the last thing someone said about me' and many others). They will then help you to challenge these thoughts and beliefs. They will set you homework tasks and help you to modify your thinking about what you are going to have a go at and about how it went when it's done. When you make some progress, they'll help you with strategies for how not to slip back.

There is evidence for efficacy of some computer-based treatments of SAD, but NICE (the National Institute for Health and Care Excellence), the national body which draws up advisory guidelines on treatment based on analysis of the research, doesn't recommend routinely suggesting computer-based treatment, so I'll leave you to discuss this with the professional from whom you're seeking treatment if the idea appeals to you.

Whatever form of therapy you engage in, give it your all and persist with it. Your life can be better than this.

Health anxiety disorder (HAD)

You have a set of symptoms which are both unpleasant and scary. You've been to your GP, had a full physical examination and appropriate blood tests. Maybe you've even seen a specialist, but no physical cause has been found for your symptoms and no diagnosis made. The natural question to ask is: 'Is it physical or psychological?' The question is natural, but it is mistaken, because the truth is that it is both. Your symptoms do have a physical basis, maybe hypersensitive sensory nerve endings, or spasm of postural muscles, or overstimulated smooth muscle in your bowels cramping up, or excessive secretion of stomach acid, or widespread overactivity of inflammatory processes, or excessive release of adrenaline and cortisol, or raised blood pressure and an elevated heart rate. Or several or all of those. All these physical changes can be the result of anxiety, and the fear they create leads to a vicious cycle.

I know this from experience. I used to suffer from atrial fibrillation (AF), a very unpleasant and potentially hazardous heart rhythm disorder. Fortunately, an operation called an 'ablation' got rid of it for me about eight years ago, but I know that at some point it may return. When I'm under stress I suffer reflux (stomach contents coming back into my oesophagus), which, in turn, causes me to suffer ectopic heart beats (I understand this is caused by distension of the oesophagus irritating the conductive tissue in the heart). These feel just like AF, which is alarming and so causes more reflux. I take a medicine which helps a bit, but what really does the trick is using CBT principles to challenge unhelpful and catastrophic thoughts (it's only palpitations and will pass), mindfulness (experience the palpitations rather than fighting them and observe them as they come and go) and relaxation (palpitations aren't incompatible with doing a relaxation exercise). As a result, the episodes, while unpleasant and a bit unsettling, are mild and transient.

There comes a point when further physical tests and appointments with specialists bear no fruit and that's the point where you should call a halt to them. But CBT and the other therapies I've listed do help. So pursue psychological therapy. This doesn't mean that you're saying your symptoms are 'all in your head'. They aren't. They are real and disabling. It means that you're pursuing a path which works, rather than continuing on along a path which is leading nowhere. If you get good at the skills listed in this book, your physical health will improve greatly and your life with it. CBT will help you to challenge the thoughts and assumptions which increase your anxiety, such as how dangerous your symptoms are, but not to challenge their physical basis, as that isn't the point. Mindfulness will help you to accept your symptoms in the present and to do less catastrophic projection about where they will lead. Your therapist will encourage you to exercise, to practise relaxation and to do whatever you would choose to do if the symptoms weren't there. Stick with the therapy; it works.

Medications which help the physical basis of your symptoms (like the medication I take to reduce my reflux) are fine but are no substitute for effective psychological therapy. Beta blockers may help if palpitations are bothersome. If you need an SSRI or something else to reduce your anxiety early in the piece, before the therapy has really worked, all well and good. Anything that works, although you'll probably be able slowly to withdraw from medication in due course.

Many people who suffer from HAD turn to alternative medicine, as they feel that conventional medicine isn't giving them the answers they need and isn't taking them seriously. Again, I have no issue with whatever works for you, but be aware that 'alternative' treatments have little evidence of efficacy and are often very expensive. If you are determined to go down the alternative route, why not do psychological therapy at the same time?

Anxiety disorders in the presence of substance misuse

Remember, alcohol reduces anxiety in the short term but, over time, it increases it. If you have become dependent on alcohol, stopping it will cause a short-term increase in anxiety. If you drink very heavily (over 50 units a week, that is 25 pints of ordinary strength beer, 17 pints of strong lager, 4 bottles of wine or two 70cl bottles of spirits a week), you should seek medical help to withdraw, as abruptly stopping on your own could be hazardous. But if you do nothing else other than stopping drinking or reducing to healthy levels (a couple of units, that is one small drink a day), your anxiety will fall over a period of one to three months back to the level it was before you started drinking to excess.

If you suffer from anxiety and alcohol dependence, you need to deal with the alcohol first, *even if the anxiety preceded and caused the drinking*. The success rate of treatments of any kind for anxiety in people who continue to drink to excess is roughly zero. On the other hand, sufferers from alcohol dependence who are success-fully treated for their addiction enjoy resolution of their anxiety in around 50 per cent of cases (even those who drank to deal with anxiety). This is probably because good addiction counselling and 12-step work as espoused by AA have a lot in common with effective anxiety treatment. Those whose anxiety doesn't resolve through addiction treatment alone subsequently tend to respond well to therapy for their anxiety. I've already explained how effective CBT, mindfulness, ACT and other therapies can be, so I won't repeat it here. Just treat your addiction first, then if you need it, get therapy for your anxiety once you're sober.

Although alcohol is probably the worst sedative drug in causing anxiety, most sedatives, if taken long term and particularly at escalating dosage, tend to have the same effect. Benzodiazepines may be an exception as they don't seem to cause worsening anxiety in those who keep at a constant low dose. The trouble is with those who increase their dose to try to abolish their anxiety. Beware chasing the illusion of an anxiety-free life with ever larger doses of sedatives. It doesn't work and will only lead to greater suffering.

If you require 'detoxification' from alcohol, that is tapering doses of medication covering the week or more following stopping drinking, the chances are that you will be given a benzodiazepine such as diazepam or chlordiazepoxide for this purpose. Don't fall into the trap of continuing this medication beyond the withdrawal period (unless your doctor has specifically advised you to). Anyone who has developed an addiction is at greatly increased risk of developing another to any potentially addictive substance, of which the benzodiazepines are all examples.

Opiate analgesics, all the way from codeine to heroin, will bring the same illusion of relief from anxiety if taken regularly and the same increase in fear and suffering over time as alcohol, but even more so. If you have become dependent on opiates, please seek treatment now. The longer you leave it, the worse it will be.

If you take stimulants such as amphetamines ('speed') or cocaine, the drug is either causing your anxiety or worsening it. All stimulants cause anxiety. Some people who take stimulants regularly become depressed after coming off them, so get in touch with your GP, who may prescribe an antidepressant to reduce this risk.

If you have suffered from any addiction, try not to fear too much what life will be like without your drug. It may be rough at first, but your future is going to be better than your past. Take it a day at a time. Some of the happiest and most serene people I have ever met have been members of Alcoholics Anonymous and Narcotics Anonymous. They are great organizations who provide help and support to so many people recovering from addiction. Google them to find a local meeting. There is no commitment, so get along to a meeting. What have you got to lose?

10

What I've learnt from patients

I hope that the last nine chapters have given you a reasonable flavour of what lies behind your anxiety, what you can do to overcome it and what treatment can offer. This is all based on fairly sound research-based evidence. But, important though research is, it isn't everything. The other important strand of evidence is the wisdom of those who have gone before, who have suffered from an anxiety disorder and found answers which worked for them. In my view, the most profound wisdom comes from those who have suffered and who have found both a meaning to their suffering and a doorway out of it. Here are some of the discoveries that my patients (and a few friends who have learnt from adversity) have shared with me, together with insights I've discovered from listening to the stories of their lives. Some have appeared earlier in this book, but I think it's worth grouping them together so that you can pick out those that you find useful.

Accept where you're starting from

This may be the most important of all insights. The main threat to you having a happy life isn't your symptoms or misfortune, it's shame preventing you from acknowledging your difficulties and doing something about them. The fact that you suffer from an anxiety disorder doesn't make you weak or worth less than the next person. Your anxiety has developed for valid reasons (see Chapter 2), which don't involve any fault of yours. In fact, anxiety disorders happen to people who I would say are among the most caring and diligent there are. I'm going to warn you against value judgements next, so I won't say that anxiety sufferers are all the best people, but they sure aren't the worst. You do need to accept that you have a problem with anxiety before you can decide on what to do about it and to get some help.

Accept who you are and try to be realistic in your aims. That is, work on reducing your cognitive dissonance (see Chapter 2).

Minimize value judgements

As I explained in Chapter 6, if you suffer from an anxiety disorder, the chances are that you're a lot more self-critical than most people. You make a lot of value judgements about yourself like 'I'm useless, feeble, pathetic, hopeless, bad, lazy, cowardly ...'. I could go on and on. This is a double standard because you're probably much less judgemental about others. If you can start to challenge these double standards, to treat yourself as you would others, your anxiety will reduce. You suffer from performance anxiety not, primarily, because you fear the judgement of others, but because you fear the judgement of *yourself*. It's *you* you're really afraid of. Sure, you dread someone criticizing you for your poor performance at whatever it is you are about to do, but that's because you've signed up to believe their criticism even before they've delivered it. So challenge this tendency. Make sure that you only say to yourself what you'd be happy to say to a good friend. Be fair and offer yourself ordinary respect.

I'm not saying that you should avoid all value judgements. You need to make some judgements about others in order to avoid surrounding yourself with people who would use and abuse you. If you lack confidence, there is a risk of you attracting these types. You also need to avoid being influenced too much by the opinions of people who don't care about you.

I recently watched the film *Denial*, about Deborah Lipstadt, who won a libel case against the Holocaust denier David

Irving. In this true story, Professor Lipstadt comments that not all opinions are of equal value. Just because someone states a contrary opinion, it doesn't mean that there are two valid sides to the argument. Opinions can be wrong if they aren't based on truth. Remember my favourite axiom: the strength of a person's opinion tends to be in inverse proportion to their wisdom. The most ignorant, bigoted and self-serving people will tend to be those who offer you the most strident opinions and advice.

Look out for these people; the ones who tell you to do what doesn't feel right. Yes, it is OK to make a judgement about them, that they are bad. That is, they are bad for you and you need to give them a wide berth.

Learn how to fail well

Anybody can succeed, at least short term. You just have to push yourself beyond human endurance. It can't last and there's a price to pay in terms of stress and wear and tear on your body, but it can be done. The really worthwhile skill is in giving it a go, giving it your all, taking a risk, sometimes coming up short, learning from your failure and treating yourself kindly while you do so. The person who can do this becomes wise and accomplished and she has no reason to be fearful. If failure is just another learning experience, there is nothing to fear. You'll have to overcome British culture to achieve this though. We've become a sadomasochistic society, hooked on punishing failure and mistakes. Just look at the newspapers after any disaster has occurred. Before the first funeral has been held, the newspapers are already baying for blood, insisting that 'someone must pay'. Whether or not anybody was guilty of malfeasance, the assumption is that if someone is punished, we'll all feel better. In truth, no good comes of the search for a scapegoat, as bad people find a way of evading responsibility, while the good ones become paralysed by fear. Don't do this to yourself. Kindness and respect are needed to learn from mistakes, particularly your own.

Some of the hardest and most important failures to embrace are failing to impress, to be liked, or to please people. Once you are able to get comfortable with not everyone liking or respecting you, you really are free. To be you and to do what *you* choose. You can then truly experience life and other people, instead of being bound up in introspective worry about how you're coming across. I can tell you from personal experience that it is incredibly liberating. Work on caring less (more on this later) and experiencing more. Develop boundaries and guard them. That is, have a good idea of what you'll agree to, what you won't and how to say no. The first time you refuse someone what they've asked of you, tolerating their disappointment and displeasure and holding your ground is the first day of your recovery. Sure, you'll feel more anxious for a while, but this fear will soon be replaced by relief. If someone has given you advice which you chose not to take, and they turned out to be right, *that's OK*. It's not wrong to be wrong sometimes, because you don't have retrospect in advance.

Act as if

This is the 'fake it to make it' tip espoused by the 12-step addiction movement, which I mentioned in Chapter 2. It works. You become the way that you act, so try acting as if you felt the way you'd like to be. Copy someone you admire. Act as if you were confident, as if it were a privilege for people to meet you, as if what you're doing is no big deal, as if you didn't care, as if the result were assured, as if panic doesn't matter. Feel the fear, but do it anyway (that's the title of a good book on overcoming phobic anxiety). Keep this going for long enough and you'll become the way you're pretending to be. This isn't dishonesty, it's practising how you want to be.

Don't walk or run on escalators

I've dealt with this in Chapter 6, but a reminder here. Let escalators, and life, take you where you're going. If the tube train is just pulling out as you reach the platform, so be it. Another train will come along. There's just as much chance of you just missing the train by standing on the escalator as there is by running down it.

There's another metaphor for this which may help. You're on a coach trip through beautiful countryside. You decide that you want to be in control of the route, so you leap out of your seat, push the driver aside and take the wheel. Oh, please, sit down! Enjoy the scenery. It may not be the scenery you chose, but it's beautiful nonetheless. If you're driving, all you'll see is the road. Release your grip on life and it'll become a lot more interesting.

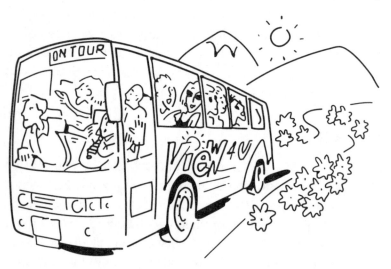

Look for opportunity, not fairness

There's a section on this in Chapter 6, so I won't repeat it all here, but don't forget it. Look out for the opportunities which come up in life and don't let pessimism cause you to avoid taking them. Take some risks …

The past doesn't predict the future

… and don't give in to superstition. The fact that you've had some bad breaks doesn't mean that you're an unlucky person who will always suffer misfortune. There is no malign imp on your shoulder making things happen. You're not under a curse. Magic only happens in the cinema and Harry Potter novels. Blow a raspberry in the face of fate. It isn't real. Worry doesn't prevent catastrophe, so it's OK to be optimistic.

Use what works for you

Everybody is different and those suffering from anxiety disorders are no exception to this rule. What helps someone else won't necessarily work for you, but something else will. Keep looking. Go through the suggestions in Chapters 5 and 6. There is an answer to your anxiety, so make sure you search until you find it. This includes anything that you want to try, not just what I've recommended. For example, if a change of diet helps, go with it. But don't waste too much time on 'alternative' treatments unless one really does it for you. And the panacea advised by your Aunt Mabel isn't likely to work, so it's OK to ignore her advice. Do listen to your treating professionals though, as there is a lot of experience and research behind their advice. If your therapist doesn't make sense for you, if it's a bad fit, ask for someone else. You may have to push for this, as resources are limited under the NHS. Everyone suffering from a severe and enduring mental disorder (if you're disabled by long-term anxiety, that includes you) is entitled to effective treatment *for them* and that doesn't mean a one-size-fits-all approach.

Reach out for support

People who have support in dealing with anxiety do much better than those who try to do it alone. Reach out to the people around you who you trust. Make sure that the people supporting you are the ones *you* choose, not necessarily the ones who choose you. Good people like to be asked. Equally though, some folks insist on you doing what they tell you, even if it isn't helpful. It can take some firmness to keep these folks at arm's length, but you need to. Surround yourself with the folks who you find healing, not those who push themselves on you.

If nothing changes, everything remains the same

This may seem obvious, but it isn't. Many people feel that if they keep doing what they've always done, things will get better. Or medication will give them a cure. This is true for situations and for individual episodes such as panic attacks (they are transient), but not for what causes them. This is one of the dangers of pharmacological treatment of anxiety. If it isn't combined with effective therapy, you may tend to wait for the medicine to cure you. It won't; instead it buys you time to make the changes you need to. Your therapist isn't going to 'make you better' either; you are, by understanding how your anxiety developed, challenging your habits and thinking, developing an action plan and acting on it. The worst thing that can happen is not what you fear, but that nothing changes. If you understand what lies behind your anxiety having read this book, start making some changes in your life now.

Care enough, but not too much

This is a really difficult balance to strike. You need to care for yourself *and* to care about others in order for them to care about you. This is something which seems to me to have been lost in the commuter belt around London. There is no sense of community or of caring about anyone other than immediate family, such is the headlong rush to success. A patient of mine, trapped standing on a packed commuter train, fainted and lay unconscious next to the door of the carriage. His fellow travellers edged away from his prostrate body but otherwise ignored him. Until the train stopped at the next station, when the two men nearest him pushed and kicked him onto the platform, being careful not to mess up their suits as they did so, and closed the carriage door behind him. Presumably these people would see themselves as civilized human beings, so what caused the moral deadness that allowed them to care so little about a fellow human being? The answer, I think, is that their anxiety about the work day which faced them and the single-minded determination required to succeed in the city of London allowed no space for compassion.

Please try to care more than this, however stressful your life and whatever threats you face. But *don't care too much*. If you worry about every person, every action, every mistake, every misfortune and every possible future, you aren't truly alive. You're living in an imaginary nightmare world of your own making, rather than experiencing the real world around you. Remember the golfer I told you about in Chapter 6, who has persuaded himself that he doesn't care about the result of his putt, only that he prepares for it and strokes it as well as he can. He became a really good putter as a result. Follow his example in running your life. Focus more on doing what you choose as well as you can, not on the result.

Why have that fantasy?

My wife, being American and like so many of her peers, had a period of therapy many years ago. She told her therapist of her many fears, to which this wise lady would usually reply, 'Why have that fantasy?' She was right. While some bad things will happen in your life, they won't be the ones you spend your time worrying about, so your worries are a total waste of time. While it may be impossible to stop worrying completely, at least get in the habit of challenging your fears, of seeing them as what they are: fantasies.

We're all going to die

A close friend of mine has metastatic prostate cancer. While he is responding very well to treatment and remains well, he is aware that one day his cancer will kill him. This remarkable man is one of the happiest and most active people I know. I asked him how he manages this in the face of an uncertain life expectancy. His reply was: 'Spoiler alert! We're all going to die. I'm going to do as much of what I love as I can before then.' Follow him, embrace your present and live it for all you're worth.

Good is better than perfect

Run your life as a marathon, not a sprint. Whether it's being good at work, parenting, fitness, health, sport, appearance or any other area of human endeavour, being consistently as good as you reasonably can be will yield better results than a search for perfection. I've treated people at the top of most occupations, rich and famous politicians, actors and sports people and, while these folks all had their problems, they all knew and accepted their limitations. I once asked a very successful professional golfer how he coped down the stretch of a major tournament, knowing that the result could change his life. He struggled to understand my question. 'You just get on and do it. You don't think beyond the next shot, or about the man you're competing against, you just hit it.' That ability to exclude everything beyond the issue immediately at hand and to do it as well as you, not someone else, can is the difference between the champions and the equally talented also-rans. So try to get better, sustainably, not perfect, not like the person you know who pretends to be a super-hero. And don't demand of yourself that you should always succeed; that isn't realistic and you wouldn't expect it of anyone else.

Deal with anger

Anger and fear are the same thing in a different form (see Chapter 1, the fight-or-flight reaction). So you need to do something about your anger if you have it, beyond just sitting on it and letting it boil. This may be through therapy, meditation, relaxation, martial arts or sublimation in work, competitive sport or exercise. But do something with it; chronic anger will hinder any efforts you make to deal with anxiety.

This too shall pass

What I'm talking about here is situations and symptoms. Your anxiety disorder is here for a while. It's likely to be a long haul, with two steps forward and one back on many occasions until it's eventually gone, if you stick with the therapy and changes you need to make.

But situations don't last. Whether it be good or bad, nothing other than love, death and taxes (yes, I borrowed that one and tweaked it) lasts forever. Wait for long enough and things will change. Your panic attack or the other physical symptoms of anxiety that are so alarming will recede in due course. So don't just do something, sit there. Don't get in the way of the natural resolution of what you're trying to escape from.

Keep going

Stick with it. It took years for your anxiety disorder to develop. Don't expect it to give up the ghost in a trice, the moment you start practising your first mindfulness exercise. It doesn't work like that. Recovery is sometimes a messy process with relapses and remissions and it's easy to become discouraged. Please don't. You remember those pop-up ads which used to plague your computer? One after another you blocked them, until eventually they stopped popping up. While spam still happens, the pop-ups have largely gone, because they can be effectively blocked given persistence. The same is true with anxiety. Stick with the therapy and the changes from this book which you implement and eventually you'll get there – a life which, while not totally free from anxiety (nobody other than the psychopath gets that), is no longer dominated by fear.

Que sera sera – Let it be

Doris Day sung the lovely song 'Que sera sera, whatever will be will be', released in 1956 (oh my goodness, I'm old!) and it made a big impression on me as a child. Whoever wrote that song knew something about psychology and, more importantly, about how to get the most out of life. Its message was that you can't dictate or even see the future, so give yourself up to it, whatever it may involve. That means your anxiety too. Don't fear your fear. Don't fight it either. Do stuff which helps and in due course overcomes your anxiety, but don't consciously fight it. When it goes, then comes back, do the same things that worked last time. If you need more therapy, get it. Do the right things, but *let your anxiety be*.

Are you feeling that this chapter is rather familiar, that it's repeating things that I've said before? Well, you're right. Welcome to psychotherapy. Overcoming your anxiety disorder is about repetition. Doing the same things over and over again. Looking at your entrenched thinking patterns from up and down and from side to side, challenging them this way and that. Changing the same tendencies over and over and over again. Your anxiety will die eventually, but it will die with a whimper, not a bang, not through any act of genius, but through repetition and plodding persistence.

You've also spotted that the therapy I delivered my patients was lifted from the wisdom of patients I'd seen before together with that of people I've been fortunate enough to bump into through my life. Oh, and the hard work of researchers and colleagues who have developed therapies that are effective. None of it was my discovery. Much of this knowledge is hundreds of years old. It's a fair cop, I'm guilty as charged. But who cares, if you can escape your fear?

Conclusion

I don't know what you think, but I reckon that much of this book is good news. You don't have to fight or struggle against your anxiety, in fact it's better if you don't. What you do matters quite a lot, but the anxiety you experience while you're doing it really doesn't, not in the short term. You don't need to feel ashamed about your anxiety disorder, in fact it suggests that you're what most people would call a good person. You don't need to be afraid of medications which, if used judiciously, are likely to help your anxiety a lot. Psychological therapies aren't scary either. They're practical, effective and their efficacy is enduring. And there's a whole load of skills you can learn and changes you can make which will not only help you to reduce your fear, but which will also improve your life in many other ways. Be patient and stick at it though. It took a long time for your anxiety disorder to develop. It's only realistic that it'll take a while for it to resolve and that there may be some reverses along the way.

So I think the time has come for us to pay another visit to Sally from the introduction to this book. I'll tell you what, why don't I sit quietly, while you talk to her? What advice are you going to give her having learnt what you have from this book? What does she need to change? What treatment should she seek and where should she start? What can she do while she's waiting for treatment to start? Have a re-read of the introduction and a think about these questions before moving on to the next paragraph. I think you know what to tell Sally and what she needs to do. It's the same as is true for you.

Now I'll tell you what I'd say to Sally. Are we on the same page? OK, here we go:

First of all Sally, *it isn't your fault*. Your anxiety disorder developed because of a combination of a bit of how you were made, but more of your life experiences, particularly early in life. You're a lovely, caring, kind person who doesn't deserve the verbal beatings you regularly dish out to yourself. Nonetheless, you are where you are now and you've got quite a lot of work to do if you're going to escape the prison which your fear has created. Accept where you're starting from and give yourself respect as you start your journey.

Next, get an appointment to see your GP. Do it now. I know getting out is almost impossible, so you'll need to have a friend or family member go with you. If you really can't get there, get a home visit from your GP. Insist, as home visits are in short supply. Get someone to phone for you if necessary. When you see your GP, tell her about your symptoms and how they've led to you being unable to get out of your flat. Ask if you need medication and take your doctor's advice on this. Most of all, ask to be referred for psychological therapy.

It's probably going to be a few weeks at least until your therapy starts. In the meantime, start practising a relaxation exercise. Get the Headspace app on your phone and try their free introductory trial. If you like it, get one of the mindfulness books I mentioned in Chapter 7. If not, try a CBT workbook. However you do it, start to challenge your habitual ways of thinking and acting. Work on accepting your anxiety rather than fighting it. Try to stay present, rather than spending so much time ruminating about the past or fantasizing about the future. Let the future, imperfections in your present, unfairness and uncertainty be. Deal with what is in front of you, not what you fear may appear. Try to change the way you speak to yourself. I don't mean out loud, but in the things you say to yourself in your head. Try to be a better friend to yourself. Being kind to yourself isn't incompatible with being kind to others; in fact, if you can start to be more charitable to yourself you'll have more kindness to give to others too. Kindness is like clover; it spreads.

And that Tricia, remind me what use she is? Yes, I know she tells you that she's wonderful and that you need her, but what does she add to your life? What, she's all you've got? Then get something or someone who is better, kinder, more giving, more reliable. I'm serious; you may think that nobody else will want to know you but they will, if you give them a chance. That means taking a risk, being lonely for a while after showing Tricia the door then, when the chance arises, interacting with someone and promising yourself that you won't judge yourself on how it goes. Success is talking to someone other than Tricia, even if they rebuff you. The result doesn't matter, just that you try. Because if you keep doing this, you'll find that some people don't rebuff you and you'll find real friends, not ones like Tricia, who only pretend to be.

You need to reach out for support to any real friends you have, the ones you've chosen, rather than those who've picked on you because they can manipulate you. The ones who listen and don't just give trite advice. The ones with real wisdom. Same with family; only confide in those who help, not those who judge. Be careful about how much support you ask for though. Seek a lot of support at the beginning, but wean yourself off gradually, becoming more self-reliant over time. If you continue to demand reassurance for everything you do, you'll become dependent on it and be unable to do anything without having your hand held.

It's going to take a while to get to the point where you can go anywhere and do anything you want. You need to start constructing your hierarchy of feared situations now, with as many rungs of as small a size as possible. No giant leaps, just one small step after another while practising relaxation as you take each rung on the ladder. No judgements about your progress or lack of it, just persistence. Accept that you'll take two steps forward and one back. Keep going and you'll get there in the end.

I'd love to be there when you get there. What a joy it will be to reveal the person you are when you get free of the fear which has hidden you for so long. In the meantime, bon voyage!

Further reading

Background

Twenge, Jean M (PhD), *iGen: Why today's super-connected kids are growing up less rebellious, more tolerant, less happy – and completely unprepared for adulthood*, Atria Books, New York, 2017.

Social anxiety disorder

Watkins, Emma, *Conversation Skills for the Shy: How to easily talk to anyone*, CreateSpace Independent Publishing Platform, 2017.

Searle, Ruth, *Overcoming Shyness and Social Anxiety*, Sheldon Press, London, 2008.

Cognitive-behavioural therapy

Bourne, Edmund (PhD), *The Anxiety and Phobia Workbook*, New Harbinger Publications, Oakland, 2015.

Mindfulness

Tolle, Eckhart, *The Power of Now*, New World Library, San Francisco, 2004.

Kabat-Zinn, Jon, *Wherever You Go, There You Are: Mindfulness meditation for everyday life*, Hyperion, New York, 2004.

Williams, Mark and Penman, Danny, *Mindfulness: A practical guide to finding peace in a frantic world*, Hachette, London, 2011.

Acceptance and commitment therapy

Hayes, Steven and Smith, Spencer, *Get Out of Your Mind and Into Your Life: The New Acceptance and Commitment Therapy*, New Harbinger Publications, Oakland, 2005.

Anxiety with depression

Cantopher, Dr Tim, *Depressive Illness: The curse of the strong*, Sheldon Press, London, 2013.

Anxiety with alcohol misuse

Cantopher, Dr Tim, *Dying for a Drink: All you need to know to beat the booze*, Sheldon Press, London, 2002.

Apps – CBT

'FearFighter' and 'SilverCloud' – Each available through GP or Mental
  Health Professional Prescription.
'Catch It' – Free for iPhone and iPad through the App Store.

Apps – Mindfulness

'Headspace' – Free for first 10 days, for Apple and Android devices.
'Calm' – Free initial trial, for Apple and Android devices.

Index